Pediatrician

International Journal of Child and Adolescent Health

Founded 1858 as 'Jahrbuch für Kinderheilkunde und physische Erziehung', continued as 'Annales Paediatrici' (1938–1966), 'Pediatric Research' (1967–1970) and 'Paediatrician' (1972–1982)

Publication data: 'Pediatrician' is published 4 times annually. Volume 12 with 4 issues appears in 1985.

Subscription rates: Subscriptions run for a full calendar year. Prices are given per volume, surface postage included.

Personal subscription: SFr. 90.–, US$44.00. (Must be in the name of, billed to, and paid by an individual. Order must be marked 'personal subscription'.)

Institutional subscription: SFr. 180.–, US$88.00. (Regular rate.)

Airmail postage: SFr. 20.–, US$11.00. (Extra per volume.)

Microform subscription: SFr. 126.–, US$61.60. (Available exclusively to subscribers of the paper edition.)

Single issues and back volumes: Information on availability and prices can be obtained through the Publisher.

Subscription orders: Orders can be placed at agencies, bookstores, directly with the Publisher S. Karger AG, P.O. Box, CH–4009 Basel (Switzerland) or with any of the following distributors:

Deutschland, West-Berlin, Ost-Europa, Naher Osten: S. Karger GmbH, Postfach 1724, D–8034 Germering/München

France: Librairie Luginbühl, 36, bd de Latour-Maubourg, F–75007 Paris

Great Britain: John Wiley and Sons, Ltd., Baffins Lane, Chichester, Sussex, PO19 1UD

USA: S. Karger Publishers, Inc., 79 Fifth Avenue, New York, NY 10003

India, Bangladesh, Sri Lanka: S. Karger India Subscription Agency, B–5/132 Safdarjung Enclave, New Delhi-110029

Japan, South Korea: Katakura Libri, Inc., 36-9 Hongo 3-chome, Bunkyo-ku, Tokyo 113

Change of address: Both old and new address should be stated and sent to the subscription source.

Bibliographic indices: This journal is regularly listed in bibliographic services.

Book Reviews: Books are accepted for review by special agreement.

Advertising: Correspondence and rate requests should be addressed to the Publisher.

KARGER

Pediatrician
Printed in Switzerland

S. Karger AG,
Postfach, CH–4009 Basel (Schweiz)

Erscheint vierteljährlich
pro Jahr 1 Band zu 4 Heften

Submission: Only original papers written in English are considered and should be sent to:

D.W. Kaplan, MD, MPH
The Children's Hospital
1056 East 19th Avenue
Denver, CO 80218 (USA)

Manuscripts should be submitted in triplicate (with three sets of illustrations of which one is an original), typewritten double-spaced on one side of the paper, with a wide margin.

Conditions: All manuscripts are subject to editorial review. Manuscripts are received with the explicit understanding that they are not under simultaneous consideration by any other publication. Submission of an article for publication implies the transfer of the copyright from the author to the publisher upon acceptance. Accepted papers become the permanent property of 'Pediatrician' and may not be reproduced by any means, in whole or in part, without the written consent of the publisher. It is the author's responsibility to obtain permission to reproduce illustrations, tables, etc. from other publications.

Arrangement:

Title page: The first page of each paper should indicate the title (main title underlined), the authors' names, and the institute where the work was conducted. A short title for use as running head is also required.

Key words: For indexing purposes, a list of 3–10 key words in English is essential.

Abstract: Each paper needs an abstract of up to 250 words.

Small type: Paragraphs which can or must be set in smaller type (case histories, test methods, etc.) should be indicated with a 'p' (petit) in the margin on the left-hand side.

Footnotes: Avoid footnotes. When essential, they are numbered consecutively and typed at the foot of the appropriate page.

Tables and illustrations: Tables (numbered in Roman numerals) and illustrations (numbered in Arabic numerals) should be prepared on separate sheets. Tables require a heading, and figures a legend, also prepared on a separate sheet. For the reproduction of illustrations, only good drawings and original photographs can be accepted; negatives or photocopies cannot be used. When possible, group several illustrations on one block for reproduction (max. size 176 × 224 mm) or provide crop marks. On the back of each illustration, indicate its number, the author's name, and 'top'. Color illustrations are reproduced at the author's expense.

References: The list of references should include only those publications which are cited in the text. References may be arranged alphabetically (citation by name and year) or numbered consecutively (citation by number).

a) Papers published in periodicals: 1. All authors' surnames ('et al.' is not sufficient) with initials of first names; 2. Full title of paper; 3. Journal abbreviation; 4. Volume (in Arabic numerals, underlined and followed by a colon); 5. First and last page; 6. Year of publication in brackets. Example: McIntosh, J.; Hansen, P.; Ziegler, J.; Penny, R.: Defective immune and phagocytic functions in uraemia and renal transplantation. Int. Archs Allergy appl. Immun. 51: 529–540 (1976).

b) Books: 1. Authors' surnames with initials of first names; 2. Full title; 3. In brackets, name and domicile of publisher and year of publication. Example: Pollack, R.S.: Tumor surgery of the head and neck (Karger, Basel 1975).

Full address: The exact postal address complete with postal code of the senior author must be given. If correspondence is handled by someone else, indicate this accordingly.

Further details: Authors may consult our leaflet 'Rules for the Preparation of Manuscripts', available on request from the Publisher, S. Karger AG, P.O. Box, CH–4009 Basel (Switzerland).

Galley proofs: Unless indicated otherwise, galley proofs are sent to the first-named author and should be returned with the least possible delay. Alterations made in galley proofs, other than the correction of printer's errors, are charged to the author. No page proofs are supplied.

Reprints: Order forms and a price list are sent with the galley proofs. Orders submitted after the issue is printed are subject to considerably higher prices. Allow five weeks from date of publication for normal delivery of reprints (airmail on request and at charge).

Diabetes in Childhood and Adolescence

29 figures, 15 tables, 1985

KARGER

Pediatrician *12:* 166–172 (1983–85)

Genetics of Insulin-Dependent Diabetes mellitus in Children

Johnny Ludvigsson

Department of Pediatrics, University Hospital, Linköping, Sweden

Key Words. Diabetes mellitus, insulin-dependent · Type-I diabetes · Genetics · Human leucocyte antigen

Abstract. Insulin-dependent diabetes in children is a heritable disease, although it does not fit into any simple genetic model. Research is not facilitated by the lack of knowledge of the different etiological mechanisms and the inability to classify the disease. Human leucocyte antigens (HLAs) coded for in the major histocompatibility complex on the 6th chromosome have given the most important insights into the genetics of diabetes, and these genes probably provide the majority of genetic susceptibility to type-I diabetes. Several facts indicate that there are at least two loci of importance, one associated with HLA B8, DR3 and another with HLA B15, DR4, which probably are usually included in extended haplotypes in linkage disequilibrium. There seems to be a substantial DNA polymorphism and further studies may detect fragments that are even more strongly associated with diabetes than the DR type. A combination of more detailed immunological, perhaps virological or other environmental investigations on diabetic patients and their families, together with the use of specific DNA probes for the HLA region, might reveal the susceptibility genes.

Diabetes is probably a polyfactorial and also a polygenic disease. The genes we trace are not always expressed phenotypically or we do not know how to discover or define phenotypes with subclinical beta-cell damage. It is therefore not surprising that it has been impossible to find a genetic model for insulin-dependent diabetes mellitus (IDDM) which easily follows the Mendelian laws.

The HLA System

Human leucocyte antigens (HLAs) coded for in the major histocompatibility complex (MHC) on the 6th chromosome (fig. 1) have given the most important insights into the genetics of diabetes. In 1974, a significant increase of the HLA types B8 and B15 was demonstrated in diabetics compared to healthy controls [1, 2]. Somewhat later a negative correlation to B7 was found and it was suggested that B7 was a protective gene [3]. Within a short time a number of studies were published showing that HLA B8 and B15, and especially if these two were combined, B8,15, were associated with an increased relative risk to develop diabetes. Rather soon an even closer connection with the DW types 3 and 4 and DW3,4 was demonstrated. This was then substituted with DR3, DR4 and DR3,4 [4, 5]. Population studies have shown that more than 90% of caucasian subjects with IDDM are positive for HLA DR3 and/or 4 haplotypes [6]. The relative risk of getting type-I diabetes in DR3,4 patients is 5–25% in different studies. The cumulative risk of getting IDDM by age 24 in HLA-identical siblings of diabetic probands has been found to be 10%, the risk for haploidentical 2.2%, and non-identical 1%. HLA identity but B7 positivity appears to protect from the effect of HLA identity [7].

Most IDDM patients bear their haplotypes in linkage disequilibrium. Three main haplotypes have been ob-

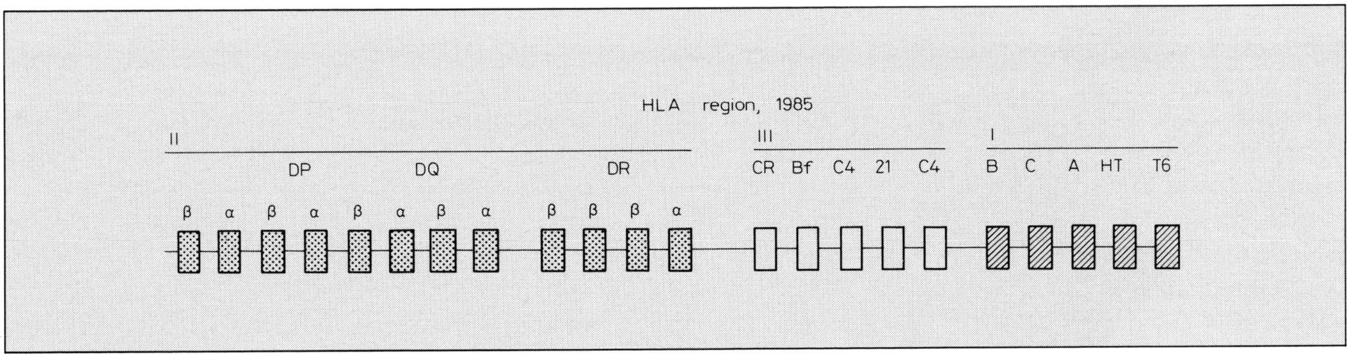

Fig. 1. The major histocompatibility complex on the 6th chromosome.

served in caucasians, two including DR3 and one DR4 [8]. It has been suggested that all of the previously described recognized increases in B8, B18, B15, DR3, DR4, etc., could be ascribed in the increase among diabetics of a few extended haplotypes such as: HLA B8, DR2; SC01; GL02; HLA B18, DR3; F1C30; HLA B15, DR4, and SC21 [9]. In fact HLA DR3 in non-extended haplotypes has been negatively related to IDDM. The data suggest that no MHC allele per se is a marker for or a suceptibility gene for IDDM, but rather extended haplotypes with relatively fixed alleles are either carriers or non-carriers of susceptibility genes for IDDM.

The HLA-D-region codes for a least three sets of products, HLA DR, HLA DQ and HLA DP, each with their own sets of alpha and beta chains [10]. By the use of specific DNA probes for the DNA region and restriction enzymes, it has been possible to show a substantial DNA polymorphism. Certain DNA fragments have been found to be increased or decreased in different individuals with the same DR type [11]. In DR4 diabetics we found a Pst 18.0-kb fragment to be increased ($p < 0.0001$) while a BamH 3.7-kb fragment was decreased ($p = 0.0003$). Genomic blotting with DNA from HLA-typed members in family studies showed that the DNA sequences were linked to HLA DR [12]. Digestion with restriction enzymes BamH1, EcoR1 dand Pst1, and hybridization with an HLA-D-region beta chain cDNA probe confirmed a BamH1 3.7-k fragment present among diabetics. A BamH1 3.2-kb fragment was found to be decreased among the diabetics compared to their non-diabetic siblings or non-related controls. BamH1 12.0-kb and 5.8-kb, EcoR1 20-kb and Pst1 6.0-kb fragments were also more frequent in diabetic individuals. Genomic blotting of DNA with a cDNA clone encoding the chain of HLA-D-region class-II antigens may improve the possibilities to detect fragments that are even more strongly associated with IDDM than the DR type. This DNA polymorphism is also pronounced in the exons and introns flanking the HLA genes. In the D region a certain polymorphism has been seen in the DQ alpha chain in contrast to the DR and DP alpha chain [13]. The variation of the DQ alpha chain may have functional significance and suggests that some aspects of the DR-associated susceptibilities could be due to variation in a DQ alpha chain. This might explain the linkage, e.g., between B15 and DR4 as a DQ alpha chain could be in linkage disequilibrium with both B15 and DR4.

B7, the suggested protective gene [3] was later substituted with DW2 and later DR2 which rarely is seen in type-I diabetics. This negative relationship may, however, just reflect a linkage disequilibrium [14].

In addition to the linkage of IDDM to the HLA markers, the properdin factor B (Bf) and glyoxalase 1 (GLO) on chromosome 6 have also been found to be associated with IDDM [15]. Thus Bfs, BfF1 and GLO seem to be positively associated with IDDM and BfF negatively [16–21].

Genes on Chromosomes Other than No. 6 Associated with IDDM

There is some evidence for the existence of other non-HLA-linked genetic loci predisposing for IDDM. A polymorphic region flanking the human insulin gene on the short arm of chromosome 11 can be described as a locus with at least three classes of alleles. A significantly higher frequency of class-I alleles and genotypes containing class-I alleles has been demonstrated in diabetic patients compared to non-diabetic controls [22]. In other studies allotypes of the Gm (immunglobulin heavy chain) locus on chromosome 14 and of Km (immunglobulin light chain) locus on chromosome 2 have been shown to be associated with IDDM [23]. Although no relationship between these allotypes and the whole group of IDDM patients has been found, a particular immunglobulin allotype, Glm (a), and a particular Gm immunglobulin phenotype (a–x–f+b+) showed a significant heterogeneity within the diabetics subdivided by HLA-DR type. Gm-associated genes could interact with these susceptibility genes at least in DR3,4 heterozygote type-I diabetics. Diabetes has also been linked to the Kid blood group located on chromosome 2 [24].

Different Modes for Inheritance of IDDM

A single locus model has been suggested. With a dominant gene [25] one would, however, expect an equal proportion of siblings sharing two or one haplotype. Furthermore the dominant single locus model does not fit with the observed distribution of HLA identical and haplo-identical siblings, and with the low frequency of IDDM among siblings (6–11%) and children (5%) of diabetics. Moreover, this model does not explain the excess of heterozygotes DR3,4. A recessive gene has also been proposed [26, 27]. However, the expected excess of DR3 or DR4 homozygotes has not been observed. In addition the frequency of IDDM among HLA-identical siblings is far less than in monozygotic twins (50%) [28] which also argues against the one locus model.

Thus, several facts indicate that there must be at least two loci of importance [21, 29], one associated with HLA B8, DR3 and another with HLA B15 DR4 [30, 31]. The class-II gene products HLA DR3 and DR4 could be the primary susceptibility genes for IDDM. They may mediate the immune mechanism which, under further influence of MHC genes class I and III, may cause diabetes. The extremely high frequency of DR3,4 heterozygotes and the genetic heterogeneity in B8, DR3 compared to B15, DR4 with regard to clinical, epidemiological and immunological parameters suggest that at least these two different susceptibility genes play an important role.

Another possibility, as mentioned above, is a model in which one or two loci located in the HLA complex and other loci on another chromosome form the genotype background, as has been suggested for the allotypes Gm or Km.

Genetic Heterogeneity of IDDM

Autoimmunity has been linked to HLA DR3 and that of susceptibility to HLA DR4 [31–33]. In patients with long IDDM duration, the prevalance of islet cell autoantibodies has been found to be higher in B8, DR3 patients than in DR4 patients [34, 35]. In a multicentre study comprising 745 HLA-DR-typed diabetic children, our earlier findings [36] that patients with DR3 have less severe clinical symptoms and signs at diagnosis and a milder early course of the disease than DR4 patients could be confirmed [37]. Other findings also suggest that genes within the human MHC control recognition and lymphocyte response to exogenous insulin components [38]. Thus, we found an association between HLA B15 and the tendency to develop insulin antibodies several years ago [3] which has been supported by other studies. There have been several attempts to correlate HLA types to the development of late vascular complications in IDDM, but no or only weak correlations have been found [39, 40]. Despite all methodological problems in studies of vascular complications, this lack of correlation to certain genes supports the view that the main cause of the vascular complications is not genetically determined but a result of the disease, i.e. the unphysiological metabolism.

Sex and Age Differences

IDDM develops more frequently in the offspring of diabetic men than in children of diabetic women [41], possibly suggesting a difference in the transmission between the sexes. However, an increased perinatal loss among diabetic mothers, and fewer children of diabetic mothers than diabetic fathers might explain this difference. Male patients have been found significantly more likely to possess DR3, while females, and also younger patients, more often possess DR4 [6, 7]. Siblings of IDDM patients, sharing two haplotypes and being relatively young at the time the proband in the family was diagnosed, had a significantly increased high risk of developing IDDM [42]. For non-HLA-identical siblings, the risk increased with increasing maternal age, which had little or no significance in HLA-identical siblings. *Deschamps* et al. [43] found similar results: the second affected sibling in families with more than one diabetic child (multiplex families) was significantly younger at the time of the proband's onset than the siblings who remained unaffected. In addition they found that the probands of multiplex families were significantly younger at onset than probands in families with a single case only. The prevalence of IDDM was higher among siblings born after than among those born before the proband. These results suggest that age-dependent factors may increase the penetrance of HLA-linked IDDM susceptibility.

Ethnic Differences

Although similar HLA associations in caucasians have been found in other ethnic groups [44, 45], there are also differences. In North American Indian patients HLA-DR3 is significantly increased and DR2 decreased, but DR4 has no significant relationship with IDDM [46]. In Korea [47] and Japan [48], B8 is rare and IDDM more associated with BW54. In Chinese children there is no relation between IDDM and B8, B15, B18, but rather a correlation to AW33, B17, BW22 [49]. Thus, there are racial differences in HLA distribution both in diabetic patients as well as in normal populations. Further genetic studies of different ethnic groups in relation to environmental factors may give important knowledge.

HLA and IDDM Susceptibility

The presence of certain HLA-associated diabetogenic genes is not sufficient to cause IDDM. Not even in pairs of identical twins is the concordance rate of IDDM more than 50%. Only up to 12–15% of diabetic patients have 1st-degree relatives with IDDM, and only about 5% of children of a diabetic parent will get IDDM before the age of 30. *Rotter and Landaw* [50] described a method estimating a 'co-efficient of genetic contribution' based on a comparison of monozygotic twin concordance data. They found that HLA genes seem to provide a coefficient of 60% for IDDM susceptibility.

Mechanisms through which HLA factors confer disease susceptibility are poorly understood. An interference with receptors on the cell surface has been suggested. *Botazzo* et al. [51] found an increased expression of class-I (HLA A, B, C) molecules in the affected islets of a diabetic patient. Some beta cells were HLA-DR-positive, however the most markedly HLA-DR-positive cells were the capillary endothelium. This together with the finding of activated (positive for HLA-DR antigen and the interleukin-2 receptor) T lymphocytes in the islets, in addition to complement-fixing IgG antibodies deposited in some islets, may give hints about the sequence of events leading to the destruction of beta cells.

Another hypothesis has been that the HLA associations just reflect the importance of other genes in the HLA region, possibly the immune-response genes. Such genes could be in linkage disequilibrium with HLA by pure coincidence and thus the HLA antigens are just secondary markers [52].

Problems with Classification

Diabetes has been regarded as the 'geneticist's nightmare' [53]. One of the reasons may be the problems with classification of the disease. For a long time it has been apparent that the manifestations of diabetes vary in different ages. In the newborn a transient form is seen but thereafter the disease has usually seemed to be chronic and irreversible. Most children get their disease rather dramatically with a short prodromal phase, while the onset in teenagers already tends to be more insidious. This form, the juvenile, in most cases is ketosis prone and totally insulin dependent, but sometimes the classical picture does not develop until after a stable period which may last for months or even years, the so-called partial remission.

In adults the rapid onset type of diabetes with total insulin deficiency is much less common. However, the number of adults with gradual onset of diabetes has increased in frequency and this type of diabetes is most common in older ages (maturity onset diabetes). The prodromal phase in maturity onset diabetes usually lasts for many years, and many of these patients never become totally insulin dependent.

Diabetes may also be divided into IDDM and the non-insulin-dependent form (NIDDM), although many patients become insulin dependent after several years of non-insulin dependency. The borderline between IDDM and NIDDM is not sharp. Thus as an example, trauma or pancreatitis can either lead to a slight insulin deficiency (NIDDM) or to a total insulin dependency (IDDM). A fracture or infection may result in insulin dependeny in a NIDDM patient, without any change in the 'diabetic disease', but as a result of an increase in metabolic stress. When modern methodology made it possible to study insulin levels, insulin sensitivity, and immunological mechanisms, it became evident that among the primary forms of diabetes one could discern different types of diabetes which had several features in common. Most IDDM patients were found to belong to type-I diabetes and NIDDM to type II [54]. Still this definition was more

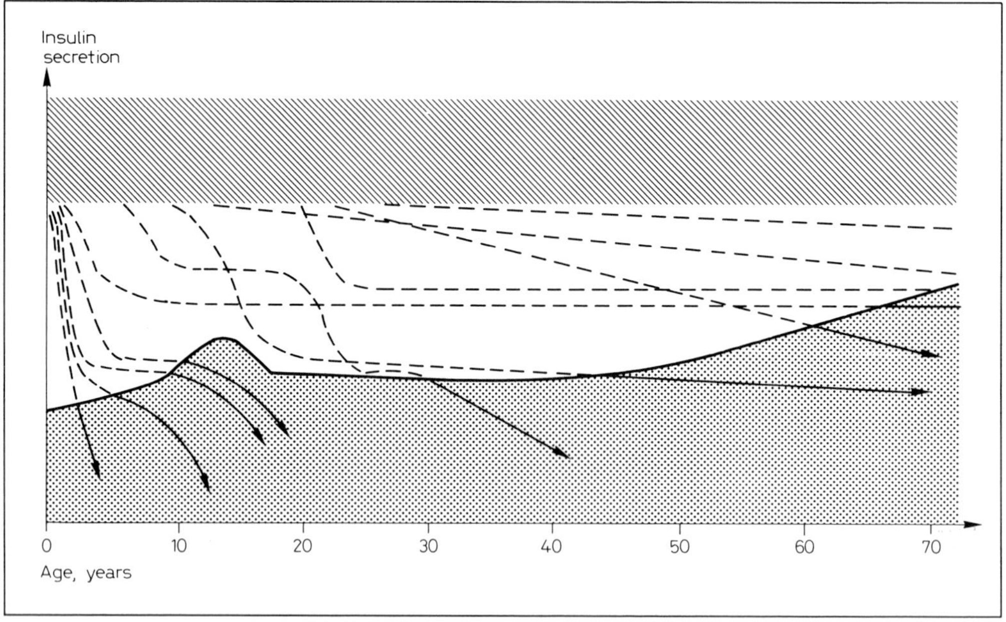

Fig. 2. After moderate damage to the beta cells enough insulin is secreted until an older age when the increased insulin requirement (because of decreased insulin sensitivity) causes manifest diabetes. ---- = Subclinical insulin deficiency; ⟶ = manifest diabetes; ▩ = insulin requirement; ▧ = optimal insulin secretion.

a definition based on course and features of the manifest disease than on etiology. Type I continued to be the earlier juvenile form even if it was accepted that type I could also be found in older ages, and a few cases of type II could be found among children.

In recent years we have learned that type-I diabetes is not necessarily the ketosis-prone IDDM with rapid onset after a short history. Many type I diabetics have a long prodromal history [55] of disturbed glucose metabolism years before diagnosis [55, 56]. When reviewing the case histories of some diabetic children, we find an atypical history of very long remissions, relapse and even repeated remissions. Furthermore, studies of type-II diabetes point at least to some similarities with type I [57].

Although the etiology, i.e. reasons for the destruction of the beta cells, certainly may vary, I would like to suggest the following possibility. Insulin requirement is low in children but increases according to growth and body weight. During puberty there is a peak and thereafter the insulin requirement decreases again. In adults it is correlated to body weight and lean body mass, but gradually increases in relation to decreased physical activity, diminished circulation, etc. (fig. 2). The totally healthy endocrine pancreas produces more insulin than needed, but in some people the islets are damaged. If this damage is very severe and early it will cause overt diabetes in childhood. In other cases a moderately damaged pancreas may produce enough insulin to fill the requirements until puberty, when the growth and hormonal imbalance will be too much for a defective pancreas. In other people with only a slightly damaged pancreas, insulin secretion may be adequate until old age when the insulin requirement becomes overwhelming. This hypothesis would presuppose that among so-called healthy people there are many with subnormal or rather suboptimal insulin secretion. Among persons with partial beta-cell damage or beta-cell disease, some of them are called type II, there may exist several damaging processes with different etiologies. In some cases an islet infection may be the cause, while in others an autoimmune process elicited by some kind of beta-cell trauma will cause the severe beta-cell loss.

As we are left to study only overt disease, i.e. the tip of the iceberg, we get an incomplete picture which forces us to talk about different degrees of genetic penetrance. We get confused since these extreme cases of beta-cell damage do not fit into any genetic model as long as the subclinical ones are missed.

Hopes for the Future

An improved knowledge of the different degrees and types of diabetes, and a combination of more detailed immunological and perhaps virological investigations of diabetic patients and their families, together with the use of DNA probes for the HLA-region genes might finally reveal the susceptibility genes. One of the DNA polymorphisms may be found to be very strongly associated with susceptibility to or protection from IDDM. Careful comparisons of ethnic groups may also add important knowledge and also give some clues why the IDDM susceptibility genes have not totally disappeared during evolution. Hopefully some day in the future the genetic code for IDDM will be identified and the etiological mechanisms clarified making it possible to prevent the manifest disease.

Acknowledgement

Our studies of genetics of IDDM in children have been supported by the Swedish Medical Council, the Swedish Diabetic Association Östergötlands County and Novo Research Institute.

References

1 Nerup, J.; Platz, P.; Ortved Andersen, O.; Christy, M.; Lyngsøe, J.; Poulsen, J.E.; Ryder, L.P.; Thomsen, M.; Staub Nielsen, L.; Svejgaard, A.: HL-A antigens and diabetes mellitus. Lancet *ii:* 864–866 (1974).

2 Cudworth, A.G.; Woodrow, J.C.: Evidence for HL-A linked genes in 'juvenile' diabetes mellitus. Br. med. J. *iii:* 133–135 (1975).

3 Ludvigsson, J.; Säfwenberg, J.; Heding, L.G.: HLA-types, C-peptide and insulin antibodies in juvenile diabetes. Diabetologia *13:* 13–17 (1977).

4 Platz, P.; Jakobsen, B.K.; Morling, N.; Ryder, L.P.; Svejgaard, A.; Thomsen, M.; Christy, M.; Kromann, H.; Benn, J.; Nerup, J.; Green, A.; Hauge, M.: HLA-D and -DR antigen in genetic analysis of insulin dependent diabetes mellitus. Diabetologia *21:* 108–115 (1981).

5 Wolf, E.; Spencer, K.M.; Cudworth, A.G.: The genetic susceptibility to type I (insulin-dependent) diabetes analysis of the HLA-DR association. Diabetologia *24:* 224–230 (1983).

6 Nerup, J.; Christy, M.; Platz, P.; Ryder, L.R.; Svejgaard A.: Aspects of the genetics of insulin-dependent diabetes mellitus; in Adreani, Immunology in diabetes (Kimpton Medical, London 1984).

7 Cavender, D.E.; Wagener, D.K.; Rabin, B.S.; Becker, D.J.; Orchar, T.J.; Eberhardt, M.S.; LaPorte, R.E.; Drash, A.L.; Kuller, L.H.: The Pittsburgh insulin-dependent diabetes mellitus (IDDM) study. HLA antigens and haplotypes as risk factors for the development of IDDM in IDDM patients and their siblings. J. chron. Dis. *37:* 555–568 (1984).

8 Dausset, J.; Hors, J.: Immunogenetics of insulin-dependent juvenile diabetes. Diab Res. *1:* 115–123 (1984).

9 Raum, D.; Awdeh, Z.; Yunis, E.J.; Alper, C.A.; Gabbay, K.H.: Extended major histocompatibility complex haplotypes in type I diabetes mellitus. J. clin. Invest. *74:* 449–454 (1984).

10 Trowsdale, J.; Lee, J.; Carey, J.; Grosveld, F.; Bodmer, J.; Bodmer, W.F.: Sequence related to HLA-Dr_a chain on human chromosome 6: restriction enzyme polymorphism detected with DC_a chain probes. Proc. natn. Acad. Sci. USA *80:* 1972–1976 (1983).

11 Owerbach, D.; Lernmark, Å.; Platz, P.; Ryder, L.; Rask, L.; Peterson, P.Å.; Ludvigsson, J.: HLA-D region B-chain differ between HLA-DR identical healthy and insulin-dependent diabetic individuals. Nature, Lond. *303:* 815–817 (1983).

12 Owerbach, D.; Hägglöf, B.; Lernmark, A.; Holmgren G.: Susceptibility to insulin-dependent diabetes defined by restruction enzyme polymorphism of HLA-D region genomic DNA. Diabetes *33:* 958–965 (1984).

13 Spielman, R.S.; Lee, J.; Bodmer, W.F.; Bodmer, J.G.; Trowsdale, J.: Six HLA-D_a chain genes on human chromosome 6: polymorphisms and associations of DC_a-related sequences with DR types. Proc natn. Acad. Sci. USA *81:* 3461–3465 (1984).

14 Platz, P.; Jakobsen, B.K.; Morling, N.; Ryder, L.P.; Svejgaard, A.; et al.: HLA-D and -DR antigens in genetic analysis of insulin-dependent diabetes mellitus. Diabetologia *21:* 108 (1981).

15 Hodge, S.E.; Anderson, C.E.; Neiswanger, K.; Sparkes, R.S.; Rimoin, D.L.: The search for heterogeneity in insulin-dependent diabetes mellitus (IDDM): linkage studies, two-locus models, and genetic heterogeneity. Am. J. hum. Genet. *35:* 1139–1155 (1983).

16 Allannic, H.; Fauchet, R.; Gueguen, M.; Pheng Savath, H.; Dinh Knoi, T.; Genetet, B.: Factor B (Bf) and glyoxalase genes in insulin-dependent diabetes mellitus. Diabète Métab. *11:* 22–26 (1985).

17 Rich, S.; O'Neill, G.; Dalmasso, A.P.; Nerl, C.; Barbosa, J.: Complement and HLA. Further definition of hih-risk haplotypes in insulin-dependent diabetes. Diabetes *34:* 504–509 (1985).

18 Rich, S.S.; Witkamp, L.R.; Barbosa, J.: Genetic heterogeneity of insulin-dependent (type I) diabetes mellitus: evidence from a study of extended haplotypes. Am. J. hum. Genet. *36:* 1015–1023 (1984).

19 Hodge, S.E.; Andersson, C.E.; Neiswanger, K.; Sparkes, R.S.; Rimoin, D.L.: The search for heterogeneity in insulin-dependent diabetes mellitus (IDDM): linkage studies. two-locus models, and genetic heterogeneity. Am. J. hum. Genet. *35:* 1139–1155 (1983).

20 Deschamps, I.; Lestradet, H.; Goderel, I.; Marcelli-Barge, A.; Schmid, M.; Hors, J.: Age-related heterogeneity of insulin-dependent diabetes mellitus. Diabète Métab. *9:* 259–263 (1983).

21 de Jongh, B.M.; Bruining, G.J.; Schreuder, G.M.; Schuurman, R.K.; Radder, J.K.; van Loghem, E.; Meera Khan, P.; Hauptmann, G.; van Rood, J.J.: HLA and GM in insulin-dependent diabetes in the Netherlands: report on a combined multiplex family and population study. Hum. Immunol. *10:* 5–21 (1984).

22 Bell, G.I.; Horita, S.; Karam, J.H.: A polymorphic locus near the human insulin gene is associated with insulin-dependent diabetes mellitus. Diabetes *33:* 176–183 (1984).

23 Schernthaner, G.; Mayr, W.R.: Immunoglobulin allotype markers and HLA DR genes in type I diabetes mellitus. Metabolism *33:* 833–836 (1984).

24 Hodge, S.E.; Anderson, C.E.; Neiswanger, K.; Field, L.L.; Spence, M.A.; et al.: Close linkage between IDDM and the Kidd blood group. Lancet *ii:* 893 (1981).

25 Spielman, R.S.; Baker, L.; Zmijewski, C.M.: Inheritance of susceptibility to juvenile onset diabetes, in Song, Skolnick, Genetic analysis of common diseases: applications to predicitive factors in coronary disease, pp. 567–585 (1979).

26 Rubinstein, P.; Suciu-Foca, N.; Nicholson, J.F.: Genetics of juvenile diabetes mellitus. A recessive gene closely linked to HLA-D and with 50 per cent penetrance. New Engl. J. Med. *297:* 1036–1040 (1977).
27 Rubinstein, P.; Grinsberg-Fellner, F.; Falk, C.: Genetics of type I diabetes mellitus: a single, recessive predisposition gene mapping between HLA.B. and Glo. Am. J. hum. Genet. *33:* 865–882 (1981).
28 Barnett, A.H.; Eff, C.; Leslie, R.D.G.; Pyke, D.A.: Diabetes in identical twins. Diabetologia *20:* 87–93 (1981).
29 Risch, N.: Segregation analysis incorporating linkage markers. I. Single-locus models with an application to type I diabetes. Am. J. hum. Genet. *36:* 363–386 (1984).
30 Cudworth, A.G.; Wolf, E.: The genetics of type I (insulin-dependent) diabetes. Curr. Probl. clin. Biochem. *12:* 45–64 (1983).
31 Bertrams, J.: The HLA association of insulin-dependent (type I) diabetes mellitus. Behring Inst. Mitt. *75:* 89–99 (1984).
32 Rotter, J.I.; Rimoin, D.L.: Heterogeneity in diabetes mellitus-update 1978: evidence for further genetic heterogeneity within juvenile onset insulin-dependent diabetes mellitus. Diabetes *27:* 599–608 (1978).
33 Cudworth, A.G.; Festenstein, H.: HLA genetic heterogeneity in diabetes mellitus. Br. med. Bull. *34:* 285–290 (1978).
34 Irvine, W.J.; McCallum, C.J.; Gray, R.S.; Duncan L.J.P.: Pancreatic islet-cell antibodies in diabetes mellitus correlated with the duration and type of diabetes, coexistent autoimmune disease, and HLA type. Diabetes *26:* 138–147 (1977).
35 Deschamps, I.; Holmberg, J.C.; Janssen, F.; Lemut, H.; Vexiau, P.; Hors, J.: Islet-cell antibodies (ICA-CFICA) and HLA genotypes in 107 IDD patients and their first-degree relatives. Hum. Immunol. *10:* 129–134 (1984).
36 Ludvigsson, J.; Lindblom, B.: HLA-DR-types in relation to early clinical manifestations in diabetic children. Pediat. Res. *18:* 1239–1241 (1984).
37 Ludvigsson, J.; Samuelsson, U.; Beauforts, C.; Deschamps, I.; Dorchy, H.; Francois, R.; Herz, G.; New, M.; Drash, A.; Schober, E.: HLA-DR 3 is associated with a more slowly progressive form of Type I diabetes. Diabetologia *29* (1986).
38 Mann, D.L.; Mendell, N.; Kahn, C.R.; Johnson, A.H.; Rosenthal, A.: In vitro lymphocyte proliferation response to therapeutic insulin components. Evidence for genetic control by the human major histocompatibility complex. J. clin. Invest. *72:* 1130–1138 (1983).
39 Sheehy, M.J.; Quintieri, F.B.; Yang, S.Y.; Alosco, S.M.; Matsui, Y.; Yunis, E.J.; Gabbay, K.H.: HLA-antigens of insulin-dependent diabetics. I. PLT colonies detecting Dw10 and a new class II determinant distinct from HLA-D. DR, MB(DC), MT, and SB. Tissue Antigens *23:* 290–300 (1984).
40 Kernell, A.; Ludvigsson, J.: Blood-retinal barriers in juvenile diabetics in relation to early clinical manifestations, HLA-DR-types and metabolic control. Graefes Arch. klin. exp. Ophthal. *222:* 250–283 (1985).
41 Warram, J.H.; Krolewski, A.S.; Gottlieb, M.S.; Kahn, C.R.: Differences in risk of insulin-dependent diabetes in offspring of diabetic mothers and diabetic fathers. New Engl. J. Med. *311:* 149–152 (1984).
42 Cavender, D.E.; Wagner, D.K.; Orchard, T.J.; LaPorte, R.E.; Becker, D.J.; Kuller, L.H.: Multivariate analyses of the risk of insulin-dependent diabetes mellitus for siblings of insulin-dependent diabetic patients. Am. J. Epidem. *120:* 315–327 (1984).
43 Deschamps, I.; Lestradet, H.; Busson, M.; Hors, J.: Evaluation of recurrence risk in siblings of diabetic children: importance of age and birth order in relation to HLA genotypes. Diabetes Res. *1:* 125–130 (1984).
44 Omar, M.A.; Hammond, M.G.; Rajput, M.C.; Asmal, A.C.: HLA A, B, C and DR antigens in young South African Indians with insulin-dependent diabetes mellitus. S. Afr. med. J. *66:* 765–767 (1984).
45 Shires, R.; Maier, G.; Lustig, A.; Barnett, P.; Joffe, B.I.; Seftel, H.C.: HLA antigens in white and black South African diabetics. S. Afr. med. J. *64:* 1087–1089 (1983).
46 Scholz, S.; Albert, E.: HLA and diseases: involvement of more than one HLA-linked determinant of disease susceptibility. Immunol. Rev. *70:* 77–88 (1983).
47 Okimoto, K.; Nakao, Y.; Matsumoto, H.; Min, H.K.; Kim, E.J.; Lee, T.H.; Yoon, J.S.; Higa, S.; Dura, T.; Mimura, G.; et al.: IgG heavy chain (Gm) allotypes and HLA-antigens in insulin-dependent diabetes mellitus in Korea. Tohoku J. exp. Med. *141:* suppl., pp. 283–287 (1983).
48 Moriuchi, J.; et al.: Association of B cell alloantigen with juvenile onset diabetes mellitus in the Japanese. Hum. Immunol. *1:* 357–362 (1980).
49 Lee, B.W.; Chan, S.H.; Tan, S.H.; Wee, G.B.; Yap, H.K.; Wong, H.B.; Tan, C.L.; Tank, K.W.: HLA-system in Chinese children with insulin-dependent diabetes mellitus: a strong association with DR3. Metabolism *33:* 1102–1105 (1984).
50 Rotter, J.I.; Landaw, E.W.: Measuring the genetic contribution of a single locus to a multilocus disease. Clin. Genet. *26:* 529–542 (1984).
51 Bottazo, G.F.; Dean, B.M.; McNally, J.M.; MacKay, E.H.; Swift, P.G.; Gamble, D.R.: In situ characterization of autoimmune phenomena and expression of HLA molecules in the pancreas in diabetic insulitis. New Engl. J. Med. *13:* 353–360 (1985).
52 Nerup, J.: HLA studies in diabetes mellitus: a review. Adv. metab. Dis. *9:* 263–277 (1978).
53 Neel, J.V.: Diabetes mellitus – a geneticist's nightmare; in Creutzfeldt, Köbberling, Neel, The genetics of diabetes mellitus, p. 1 (Springer, Berlin 1976).
54 Cudworth, A.G.: Type I diabetes mellitus. Diabetologia *14:* 281–291 (1978).
55 Gorsuch, A.N.; Lister, S.; Dean, B.M.; Spencer, K.M.; McNally, J.M.; Botazzo, G.F.; Cudworth, A.G.: Evidence of a long prediabetic period in type I diabetes mellitus. Lancet *ii:* 1363–1365 (1981).
56 Rossini, A.A.; Mordes, J.P.; Like, A.A.: Animal models of insulin-dependent diabetes mellitus; in Andreani, Federlin, Di Mario, Heding, Immunology in diabetes (Kimpton Medical, London 1984).
57 Cerasi, E.: A la recherche du temps perdu – epilogue to the Minowski Award lecture 1974. Diabetologia *28:* 547–555 (1985).

Received: January 28, 1986

Johnny Ludvigsson, MD,
Department of Pediatrics,
University Hospital,
S–581 85 Linköping (Sweden)

Pediatrician *12:* 173–178 (1983–85)

0300–1245/85/0124–0173$2.75/0

Immunologic Aspects of Type I Diabetes

Michael J. Dobersen, H. Peter Chase

Department of Pediatrics, University of Colorado Health Sciences Center, Barbara Davis Center for Childhood Diabetes, Denver, Colo., USA

Key Words. Diabetes · Immunology · Islet cell antibodies · Insulitis · Cyclosporine

Abstract. Accumulating evidence supports the theory of an immunologic component in type I diabetes. The serum islet cell antibodies, the increased number of Ia-positive T cells in the peripheral blood of some new-onset patients, the presence of inflammatory cells in the islets and the apparent response of patients with new-onset diabetes to immunosuppressant medications all lead to this conclusion. However, it is still unknown if the immunologic aspects of the disease are primary or secondary phenomena. This question aside, it will be necessary to understand the immunologic factors if transplantation is to be successful as a permanent cure. If these factors are not understood and controlled, they will likely again result in destruction of the newly transplanted islet tissue. It is also probable that an understanding of the ongoing immunologic damage in the prediabetic stage will be necessary if diabetes is to be prevented. Clearly, much more research related to the immunologic aspects of type I diabetes is needed.

Introduction

Evidence has increased in recent years to suggest that insulin-dependent diabetes mellitus (type I diabetes) has an immunologic component. It is unknown, however, if the immunologic component is secondary to damage caused by another agent(s), or if it is a primary phenomenon. The issue is further confused by the likelihood that type I diabetes represents a group of disorders which may have a similar mode of presentation. It would seem likely that in most cases a genetic predisposition allows a viral, chemical or other mechanism to initiate damage to the islet cells. A secondary immunologic process may then be responsible for the ongoing destruction of the islets (fig. 1). This review of the immunologic factors that are thought to be related to type I diabetes will be divided into: (1) islet cell antibodies, (2) changes in peripheral blood lymphocytes, (3) pancreatic inflammation and (4) the use of immunosuppressive medications to delay the onset of type I diabetes.

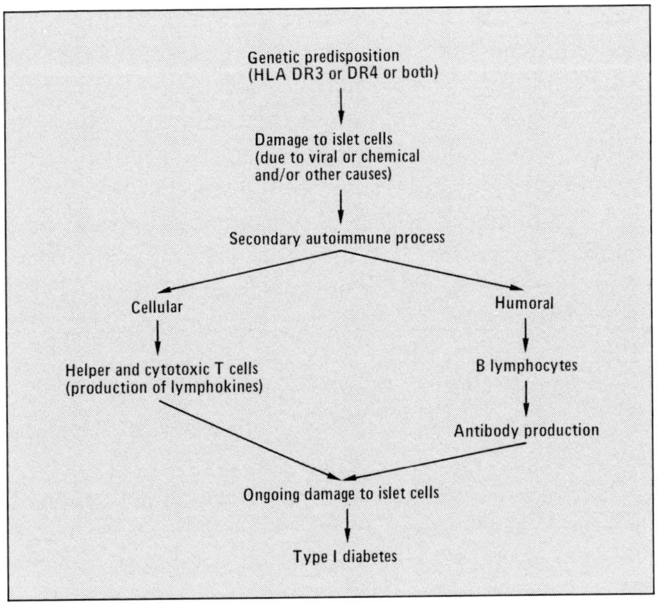

Fig. 1. Possible interrelationships between pathogenic factors associated with the development of type I diabetes.

Islet Cell Antibodies

It has been known for many years that islet cell antibodies (ICAs) were present in the serum of 70–90% of patients with new-onset type I diabetes [1, 2]. These are commonly referred to as 'cytoplasmic' because they cause staining of the cytoplasm of the islet cells (fig. 2). They are an IgG antibody. The ICA test is positive for people with type I diabetes but not for people with type II diabetes. Interest has peaked recently with the realization that serum antibodies may be present for many years prior to the onset of type I diabetes [3, 4]. In one study of 24 pairs of identical twins in which the first twin developed type I diabetes mellitus, three discordant twins had islet cell antibodies for 5, 7 and 8 years prior to the onset of type I diabetes [4]. In a prospective study of first degree relatives of people with type I diabetes, sixteen of 1,723 (0.9%) had ICAs [5]. Two of the 16 relatives with ICAs and 1 of the 1,707 relatives without ICAs developed diabetes over a maximum follow-up period of 2 years.

A major problem with the ICA test is that the results vary greatly between laboratories. The test is a fluorescent antibody reaction in which the patients' serum is incubated with fluorescein and with frozen sections of blood group O human pancreas. Group O pancreas glands are required to prevent interfering staining of the acinar pancreas from expression of blood group antigens. The sensitivity of the assay can be improved by the use of a longer incubation time (24 h) with aprotinin added to the buffer to prevent the action of pancreatic digestive enzymes [6]. It is likely, however, that the selection of the type O human pancreas is the most important parameter in determining the sensitivity of the assay. Some pancreases result in a good staining reaction while others do not. Regardless, the assay depends on a subjective microscopic reading of the amount of fluorescence present.

A recent paper described the target antigen to be a sialoglycoconjugate [7]. If the antigen clearly can be identified and then be produced in adequate quantity, it is likely that a more accurate assay will be developed. This probably would be either an enzyme-linked immunosorbent assay (ELISA) or a radioimmunoassay which would then allow the screening of large populations at relatively low cost.

Table I presents the results of screening patients with new-onset type I diabetes in 1984–1985 in our clinic. Ninety percent of the new-onset patients had ICAs at the onset. Two boys who had ICAs prior to the onset of the diabetes were negative at the time of beginning insulin therapy. We have found it to be common for the antibody levels to fluctuate – even to the point of being intermittently negative, prior to the onset of the diabetes. This is true even when multiple samples drawn from the same patient at different times are run simultaneously. The variability in staining may represent different degrees of pancreatic damage occurring during the prediabetic state.

Table I. Presence of cytoplasmic ICAs at the time of diagnosis in children and adolescents with new-onset type I diabetes

ICA test result	Number of people	Percentage
Strongly positive	26	36.5
Positive	26[1]	36.5
Weakly positive	12[1]	17
Negative	7[2]	10

1 Includes 1 person with diabetes developing secondary to cystic fibrosis.
2 Includes 2 people who were positive for ICAs in the prediabetic period, but who were negative at the time of starting insulin treatment.

Also included in table I are results from two patients with cystic fibrosis who had ICAs at the time of diagnosis. This has not been reported previously and provides further evidence that the ICAs are a secondary phenomenon and not the initiating factor in causing diabetes. Patients with cystic fibrosis have thick secretions which block the pancreatic ductules causing a secondary increase in pressure and loss of the acinar tissue. Eventually the islet cell tissue also is damaged and diabetes results. There is no relationship of the diabetes in patients with cystic fibrosis to DR typing [8]. Both of our patients with cystic fibrosis who developed diabetes had ICAs present in their serum. The damage to the islets from the back up in pancreatic secretions clearly was the cause of the ICAs and the diabetes. Thus, the ICAs were a secondary phenomenon and not the primary cause of the diabetes.

In addition to the standard cytoplasmic IgG ICAs discussed above, there are several other types of cytoplasmic antibodies which also may be important. *Gorsuch* et al. [3] found the cytoplasmic IgG antibody to be present in the prediabetic phase in 6 of 582 first degree relatives of people with type I diabetes. All six eventually became diabetic. However, he also found a second cytoplasmic antibody detected by complement fixation that was positive in 5 of the 6 during the prediabetic phase. The relation between the complement-fixing antibody and the

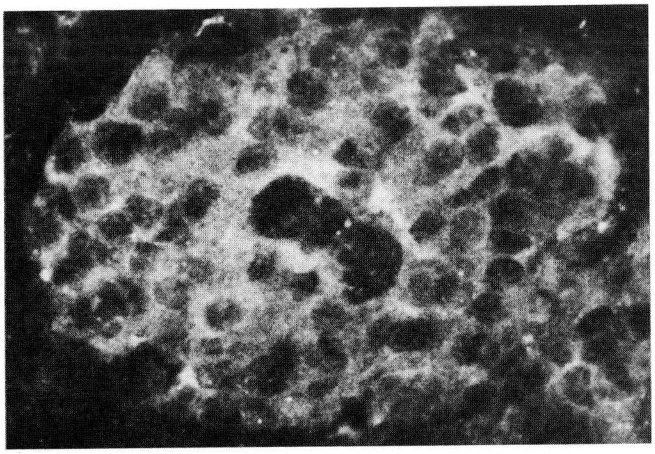

Fig. 2. Photomicrograph of positive fluorescent cytoplasmic ICA test using serum from child with new-onset diabetes and cryostat section of normal group O human pancreas. Note the diffuse staining of the cytoplasm.

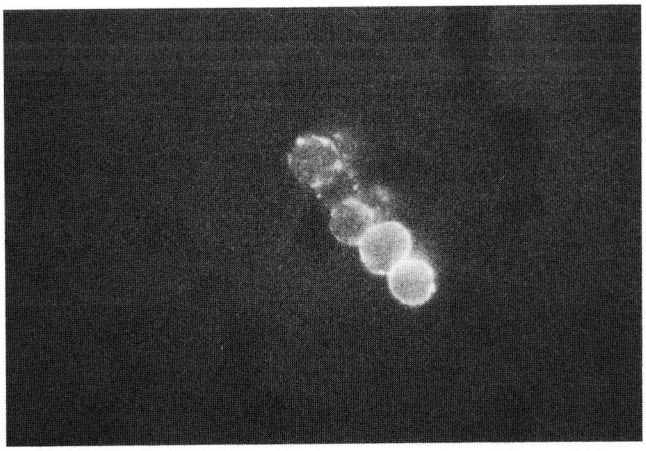

Fig. 3. Photomicrograph demonstrating islet ICSA. Serum from a child with new-onset type I diabetes was incubated with a suspension of newborn rat islet cells. The ICSA binding was demonstrated by an indirect immunofluorescent technique [10]. Note the staining primarily on the cell surfaces.

conventional IgG antibody remains to be elucidated; however, they do seem to represent distinct entities. A recent review [9] included discussion of other ICAs which stain the cytoplasm of the islet cells only on Bouin's fixed human pancreas. These antibodies may be different from both the conventional IgG antibody and the complement-fixing antibody. Future studies are required to ascertain the similarities and differences between these antibodies.

In addition to the cytoplasmic ICAs, another type of antibody has been found which is detected only on the surface of the β-cell; these are referred to as islet cell surface antibodies (ICSAs). ICSAs can be detected in human serum by indirect immunofluorescence (fig. 3) using any one of several types of islet cells (mouse, rat, rat islet monolayer cultures or human β-cells) as the substrate [9]. A radioactive chromium release double-fluorescence cytotoxicity assay is now often used for ICSA detection [10]. The ICAs and the ICSAs are usually found concurrently in new-onset diabetics [11]; however, it is likely that the two are separate antibodies.

Unlike ICAs, the ICSAs appear to be β-cell-specific. Using the double-fluorescence cytotoxicity assay mentioned above, it has been shown that while rat β-cells were readily lysed by ICSAs and complement, the other islet cell types were spared [12]. While it is not known whether ICSAs are directly pathogenic or a reflection of β-cell damage, their cytotoxic nature is consistent with a role as a primary mediator of immune damage. Further, the demonstration that these antibodies are preferentially lytic for β-cells may be one of the explanations for the selected loss of these cells in patients with type I diabetes.

Changes in Peripheral Blood Lymphocytes

The spontaneously diabetic BB rat, considered one of the best experimental models for human type I diabetes, has severe reductions in peripheral blood lymphocytes [13]. This lymphopenia occurs in animals that become diabetic as well as in animals that do not develop diabetes. It is mainly due to a reduction in T lymphocytes, with the helper/inducer subset reduced the most, and the other subsets being less affected. The evidence for similar changes in the human with new-onset type I diabetes is less convincing.

The only confirmed alteration of lymphocyte phenotype in people with type I diabetes is an increased number of T lymphocytes bearing the Ia antigen [14]. This antigen is coded for by the HLA-D region of chromosome 6 and is normally present on all B lymphocytes and some monocytes, but not in large amounts on normal T cells unless they are activated. Murine monoclonal anti-Ia antibody L243 was used in the study and reacts with a nonpolymorphic region of the Ia antigen. Nine of eleven patients with type I diabetes for less than 6 months had more than 7% Ia-positive T cells; controls and patients with type II diabetes had less than 1.5% Ia-positive T cells.

A number of other diseases which are considered to have an immunologic component, including rheumatoid arthritis, infectious mononucleosis and systemic lupus erythematosus are also associated with an increased number of Ia-positive T cells [15]. Patients with Graves' disease also have an elevation in the number of T lymphocytes bearing the Ia antigen [16]. Unfortunately, any recent infection also may cause an increase in activated T cells. As it is common for patients with type I diabetes to have an acute infection as the final insult at the time of developing diabetes, it is not impossible that the increased number of activated T cells are secondary to an infection.

A recent study used a direct immunofluorescence technique on whole blood followed by flow cytometry analysis [17]. This avoided technical artifacts that Ficoll-Hypaque flotation and rosetting with sheep red blood cells might introduce. Patients with type I diabetes were divided into group 1 (duration of diabetes of 0–1 month), group 2 (duration of 1 month–4 years), group 3 (duration >4 years) and group 4 (controls). There were no statistically significant alterations in the T cell subpopulations in the newly diagnosed patients (group 1) although 4 of 14 patients showed a percentage of activated T cells higher than the mean ± 2 SD of the controls. Total lymphocyte count also was not altered. Only group 2 patients showed a significant increase ($p < 0.05$) in the activated T cells. Surprisingly, only group 3 patients showed a mild lymphopenia.

In contrast to the BB rat and NOD mouse which develop spontaneous diabetes and have lymphopenia, there are no consistent lymphocyte alterations in people who develop type I diabetes. Further studies will be necessary to determine the significance and role of T cell activation. Is it primarily related to being HLA/DR3-positive (as suggested by *Pozzilli* et al. [18] in a study of healthy first degree relatives of type I patients)? Is it related to infections present at the clinical onset of diabetes? Is there a specific relationship to an autoimmune process occurring in these patients? More research will be necessary in order to answer these questions.

Pancreatic Inflammation

The concept of an autoimmune component in type I diabetes was initially suggested by the presence of inflammatory lesions, termed 'insulitis' in the pancreatic islets of some people with new-onset diabetes [19]. Insulitis occurs in at least 70% of patients with type I diabetes of less than 6 months duration [19–22]. Photomicrographs demonstrate a normal pancreas (fig. 4) and the acute (fig. 5) and the chronic (fig. 6) inflammation occurring with the diabetic process. Chronic inflammation can be identified in islets with normal-appearing cells as well as in islets that have been totally depleted of β-cells; acute inflammation is rarely seen. Frequently there is evidence of regeneration of islet cells, particularly β-cells. After a year of diabetes, the islets appear histologically atrophic because of the absence of β-cells although the remaining islet cells are fully granulated with their respective hormones. At this time there is no evidence of inflammation.

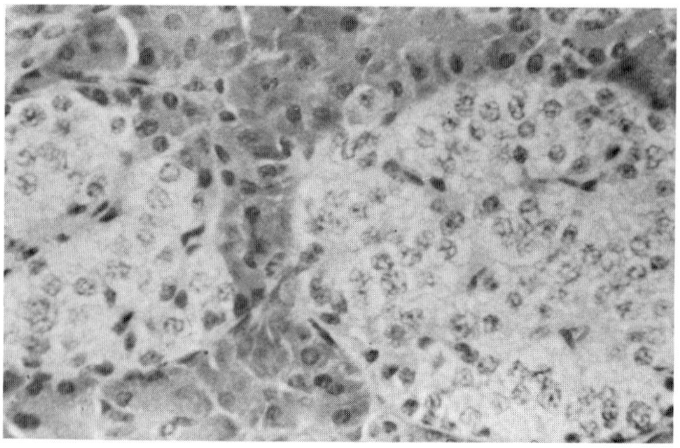

Fig. 4. Normal human islets. HE. × 2,000.

Of particular interest is the striking specificity of the immune attack against the insulin-producing β-cell. At least three other cell types are present in the pancreatic islets (glucagon-producing α-cells, somatostatin-producing δ-cells and pancreatic polypeptide-producing PP cells). Analysis of islets from patients with IDDM as well as from experimental diabetic animals indicates that only the β-cells are destroyed with a general sparing of the other islet cell types.

The types of lymphocytes found in the pancreas at the time of diagnosis are primarily cytotoxic/suppressor T cells [22]. Similar cell types have also been found around the thyroid follicles in autoimmune thyroiditis [23]. *Bottazzo* et al. [22] described some of the T cells in the pancreas to be 'activated' (positive for HLA-DR antigens and the interleukin-2 receptor). They also found immunocytes bearing IgG scattered in the pancreas and comple-

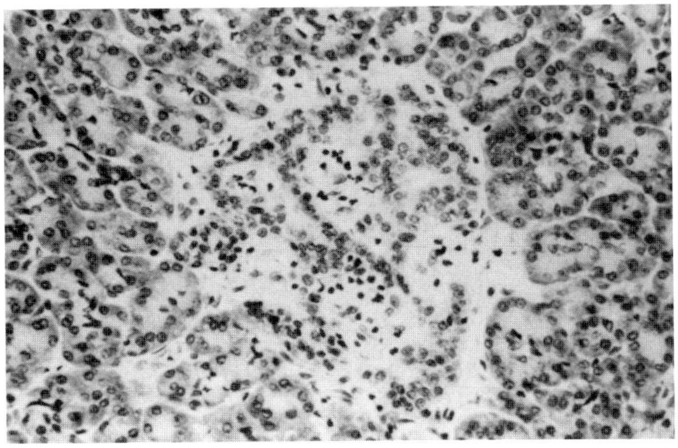

Fig. 5. Acute inflammation of islet cell (insulitis) from a child dying of new-onset diabetes. Note disruption of general architecture of the islet with remaining cells organized into cords. Also present are numerous infiltrating mononuclear cells. HE. × 1,250.

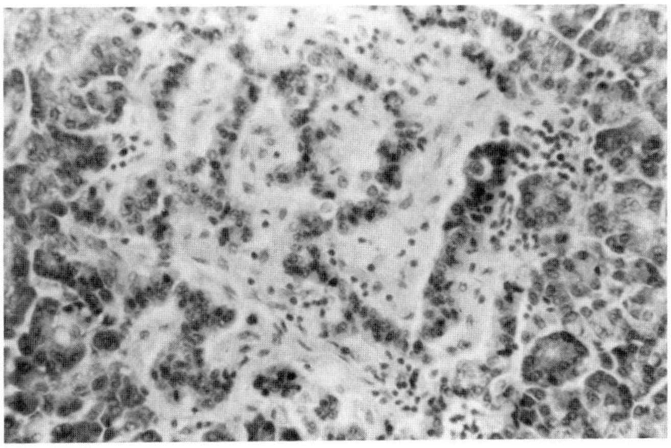

Fig. 6. Chronic inflammation of an islet from a child dying approximately 4 weeks after diagnosis of type I diabetes. The disruption of architecture, cording of remaining tissue and growth of fibrous tissue are evident. Mononuclear cells are less evident HE. × 1,250.

ment-fixing IgG antibodies deposited in some islets. These findings strongly support the role for an immunologic component in the etiology of type I diabetes.

Immunosuppression and Type I Diabetes

Cyclosporine [24] and most other immunosuppressant medications tested have been shown to prevent diabetes in the BB rat. It is argued that if an immunosuppressant medication can prevent the disease, there must be an immunologic component in the etiology. However, as noted earlier, the disease in both animal models (BB rat and NOD mouse) is different from human diabetes. Because of the animal research and because of other evidence relating diabetes to an immunologic disorder, numerous immunosuppressant medications have been or are now being tried in humans with new-onset type I diabetes [25]. A Canadian study has reported the greatest success to date after giving cyclosporine to people within 6 weeks of onset of type I diabetes [26]. Sixteen of thirty patients 'became insulin independent with concentrations of plasma C-peptide in the normal range and decreasing titers of islet cell antibodies' while receiving the medication. Unfortunately, the study was not controlled and it compared the remission rate with a previous study in which the remission rate was not tested, but in which the rate was stated to be approximately 3%. A second study from France [27] described the use of cyclosporine in 12 recently diagnosed patients with type I diabetes. Four patients (33%) had a complete remission and the insulin needs of four more were cut by half. A nonrandomized control group was reported to have an incidence of remission of 6%. Although these studies appear encouraging, they lack proper control groups. The mechanism of action of cyclosporine is uncertain. It is currently believed to act by suppressing T lymphocyte production of lymphokines, which are essential for differentiation of those lymphocytes into activated forms (e.g. cytotoxic T lymphocytes) [28]. Cyclosporine has been the most effective immunosuppressant to date in preventing the rejection of allografts. Unfortunately, it also has very serious side effects which include possible renal damage [29] and/or carcinogenic activity. The effect in patients with new-onset diabetes occurs only during the period of treatment; cyclosporine is not a medication to give indefinitely unless necessary to sustain life. Thus, safer agents which may be able to be given for life must be found and investigated. The Canadian study concluded: 'The results of our study support the theory of an autoimmune pathogenesis for type I diabetes' [26]. However, until properly controlled studies are completed, this conclusion may be premature. Currently, cyclosporine is not recommended for the treatment of new-onset patients with type I diabetes except in properly controlled research studies.

Acknowledgement

This work was supported in part by a grant (RR69) from the General Clinical Research Centers Program of the Division of Research Resources, National Institutes of Health.

References

1 Lendrum, R.; Walker, G.; Cudworth, A.G., et al.: Islet cell antibody in diabetes mellitus. Lancet *ii:* 1273–1276 (1976).

2 Bottazzo, G.F.; Gorsuch, A.N.; Dean, B.M., et al.: Complement-fixing islet-cell antibodies in type I diabetes: possible monitors of active beta cell damage. Lancet *i:* 668–672 (1980).

3 Gorsuch, A.N.; Lister, J.; Dean, B.M., et al.: Evidence for a long prediabetic period in type I (insulin dependent) diabetes mellitus. Lancet *ii:* 1363–1365 (1981).

4 Srikanta, S.; Ganda, O.P.; Jackson, R.A., et al.: Type I diabetes mellitus in monozygotic twins: chronic progressive beta cell dysfunction. Ann. intern. Med. *99:* 320–326 (1983).

5 Srikanta, S.; Ganda, O.P.; Rabizadeh, A., et al.: First-degree relatives of patients with type I diabetes. Islet cell antibodies and abnormal insulin secretion. New Engl. J. Med. *313:* 461–464 (1985).

6 Pilcher, C.; Elliott, R.B.: Improved sensitivity of islet cell cytoplasmic antibody assay in diabetics. Lancet *i:* 1352 (1984).

7 Nayak, R.C.; Omar, M.A.K.; Rabizadeh, A., et al.: 'Cytoplasmic' islet cell antibodies. Evidence that the target antigen is a sialoglycoconjugate. Diabetes *34:* 617–619 (1985).

8 Schwarz, H.P.; Bonnard, G.D.; Neri, T.M.: Histocompatibility antigens in patients with cystic fibrosis and diabetes mellitus. J. Pediat. *104:* 799–800 (1984).

9 Dobersen, M.J.: Humoral autoimmune aspects of insulin-dependent (type I) diabetes mellitus. Concepts Immunopathol. *2:* 47–64 (1985).

10 Dobersen, M.J.; Scharff, J.E.; Ginsberg-Fellner, F., et al.: Cytotoxic autoantibodies to beta cells in the serum of patients with insulin-dependent diabetes mellitus. New Engl. J. Med. *303:* 1493–1498 (1980).

11 Lernmark, A.; Hagglof, B.; Freedman, Z.R., et al.: A prospective analysis of antibodies reactive with pancreatic islet cells in insulin-dependent diabetic children. Diabetologia *20:* 471–474 (1981).

12 Dobersen, M.J.; Scharff, J.E.: Preferential lysis of pancreatic beta cells by islet cell surface antibodies. Diabetes *31:* 459–462 (1982).

13 Yale, J.F.; Grose, M.; Marliss, E.B.: Time course of the lymphopenia in BB rats. Relation to the onset of diabetes. Diabetes *34:* 955–959 (1985).

14 Jackson, R.A.; Morris, M.A.; Haynes, B.F., et al.: Increased circulating Ia-antigen-bearing T cells in type I diabetes mellitus. New Engl. J. Med. *306:* 785–787 (1982).

15 Winchester, R.J.; Kunkel, H.G.: The human Ia system. Adv. Immunol. *28:* 221–292 (1979).

16 Jackson, R.A.; Haynes, B.F.; Burch, W.M.; Shimizu, K.; Bowring, M.A.; Eisenbarth, G.S.: Ia positive T cells in new onset Graves' Disease. J. clin. Endocr. Metab. *59:* 187–190 (1984).

17 Pontesilli, O.; Chase, H.P.; Carotenuto, P., et al.: T-lymphocyte subpopulations in insulin dependent (type I) diabetes mellitus. Clin. exp. Immunol. *63:* 68–72 (1986).

18 Pozzilli, P.; Sense, M.; Al-Sakkaf, L., et al.: Prospective study of lymphocyte subsets in subjects genetically susceptible of type I (insulin-dependent) diabetes. Diabetologia *27:* 132–135 (1984).

19 Gepts, W.: Morphological pathology of the islets of Langerhans in juvenile diabetes; in Etiology and pathogenesis of insulin-dependent diabetes mellitus, pp. 1–12 (Raven Press, New York 1981).

20 LeCompte, P.M.; Gepts, W.: The pathology of juvenile diabetes; in Volk, Wellman, The diabetic pancreas, p. 325 (Plenum Press, New York 1977).

21 Gepts, W.: Pathologic anatomy of the pancreas in juvenile diabetes mellitus. Diabetes *14:* 619–633 (1965).

22 Bottazzo, G.F.; Dean, B.M.; McNally, J.M., et al.: In situ characterization of autoimmune phenomena and expression of HLA molecules in the pancreas in diabetic insulitis. New Engl. J. Med. *313:* 353–360 (1985).

23 Bene, M.-C.; Derennes, V.; Faure, G., et al.: Graves' disease: in situ localization of lymphoid T cell subpopulations. Clin. exp. Immunol. *52:* 311–316 (1983).

24 Laupacis, A.; Gardell, C.; Dupre, J., et al.: Cyclosporin prevents diabetes in BB Wistar rats. Lancet *i:* 10–12 (1983).

25 Rossini, A.A.: Immunotherapy for insulin-dependent diabetics? New Engl. J. Med. *308:* 333–335 (1983).

26 Stiller, C.R.; Dupre, J.; Gent, M., et al.: Effects of cyclosporine immunosuppression in insulin-dependent diabetes mellitus of recent onset. Science *223:* 1362–1367 (1984).

27 Assan, R.; DeBray-Sachs, M.; Laborie, C., et al.: Metabolic and immunological effects of cyclosporin in recently diagnosed type I diabetes mellitus. Lancet *i:* 67–71 (1985).

28 Bunjes, D.; Hardt, C.; Kollinghoff, M., et al.: Cyclosporin A mediates immunosuppression of primary cytotoxic T cell responses by impairing the release of interleukin 1 and interleukin 2. Eur. J. Immunol. *11:* 657–661 (1981).

29 Myers, B.D.; Ross, J.; Newton, L., et al.: Cyclosporine-associated chronic nephropathy. New Engl. J. med. *311:* 699–705 (1984).

Received: December 6, 1985

H. Peter Chase, MD,
Department of Pediatrics,
University of Colorado Health Sciences Center,
Barbara Davis Center for Childhood Diabetes,
4200 East 9th Avenue,
Box B-140,
Denver, CO 80262 (USA)

Pediatrician *12:* 179–193 (1983–85)

0300–1245/85/0124–0179$2.75/0

Insulin-Dependent Diabetes: A Possible Viral Disease

Giuseppe Saggese[a], *Giovanni Federico*[a], *Carlo Garzelli*[b], *Antonio Toniolo*[b]

[a] Department of Pediatrics and [b] Institute of Microbiology, University of Pisa, Italy

Key Words. Insulin-dependent diabetes · Viruses · Epidemiology · Pathogenesis · Autoimmunity

Abstract. The available information regarding the possible relevance of viruses in the pathogenesis of insulin-dependent diabetes is reviewed. Experimental studies in animals, clinical cases, histopathologic findings as well as epidemiologic and family studies provide circumstantial evidence that at least some cases of the disease are triggered by infection. Moreover, since it is widely accepted that autoimmunity plays a key role in diabetogenesis, the possible relationship between viruses and the induction of autoimmune responses to pancreatic islets is discussed. In view of recent developments in our comprehension of several chronic 'idiopathic' diseases, the role of persistent viral infections and virus-induced immunopathology deserve further consideration in the etiology and pathogenesis of diabetes.

Introduction and Epidemiologic Aspects

Over the last decade, the recognition of new immunologic and genetic markers has allowed the distinction of at least three pathogenetic forms of insulin-dependent diabetes mellitus (IDDM) which are thought to derive from different insults to beta cells: (1) organ-specific autoimmunity, (2) a mixture of autoimmune and environmental factors and (3) environmental factors alone [1]. Recent epidemiologic, immunologic and pathologic studies clearly suggest that a long prediabetic period of several months up to a few years precedes the onset of the disease in most cases [2]. This new concept makes investigations on the causes of the disease obviously more difficult, since it is extremely hard to uncover cause-effect relationships on a long-time scale.

However hard the problem can be, as in other chronic human diseases, epidemiologic analysis and family studies have shed some light upon the role of genetic factors and of environmental influences in the etiology of IDDM. Most notably, the studies of *Pyke* [3] on monozygotic twins have shown that IDDM is present in both probands only in about half of the cases and careful studies indicate that unaffected twins are normal, not prediabetic. These observations, confirmed by others, indicate that genetic factors certainly predispose to IDDM, but that they are not sufficient by themselves in causing the disease. Thus, it appears that the exposure to unknown diabetogenic agents is an absolute prerequisite for the development of IDDM.

Though experimental work on animals has shown that diabetogenesis can be promoted by both chemical and viral agents [4, 5], the available evidence derived from epidemiologic patterns seems more compatible with an infectious etiology rather than with a toxic one:

(1) Infants under nine months are usually spared, as is seen with many viral diseases where maternal antibodies confer passive protection;

(2) All over the world the incidence peak is between 10 and 15 years of age, and onset after 35 years is exceptional;

(3) In pairs of siblings where both are diabetic, the interval between onsets is usually shorter than 1 year, as if the causative agent had a relatively short period of action;

(4) There is a clear-cut seasonal cycle peaking between December and March in Northern Europe and in the United States. *Gamble* [6] observed that in the United Kingdom the peak is quite consistent from year to year and the peak incidence is about twice the trough incidence. The seasonality is more prominent in children

under age 6 than in older patients. These observations are consistent with the proposal that the onset of IDDM is preceded by a triggering event, such as a virus infection which has a seasonal distribution (fig. 1A). It is also noteworthy that in Chile and in Melbourne (i.e., in the Southern hemisphere) the seasonality of IDDM is 6 months offset from this cycle. This same phenomenon is characteristic of conventional virus infections such as mumps and enteroviral diseases (fig. 1B).

Although the generally seasonal occurrence of IDDM has been observed worldwide, new cases develop throughout all months of the year. This suggests that if there is an association between viral infections and diabetes it is complex: for instance, the development of diabetes might require cumulative insults to beta cells or derive from infections with long-acting diabetogenic viruses.

An association of diabetes and antecedent mumps virus infections was noted as early as 1864 by the Norwegian physician *J. Stang,* in 1899 by *Harris* in the US, and in 1924 by *Gundersen* who reported that epidemics of parotitis in Norway at the beginning of this century were followed by 4-year periods during which there was an increased number of deaths due to juvenile diabetes [7]. Epidemiologic studies performed more recently in New York State and in Sweden led to the same conclusion. Taken together, these studies suggest that diabetes may develop a few months to 4 years after mumps infection. However, a recent study of *Gamble* [8] indicates that epidemiologic links between clinical parotitis and diabetes can be found only in a few percent of cases.

Diabetes has also been reported to follow an epidemic of infectious hepatitis in Nigeria, and sporadic reports suggest a possible link with other viral diseases such as infectious mononucleosis, influenza and coxsackie B infections. However, the only firm epidemiologic connection between viruses and IDDM refers to the congenital rubella syndrome.

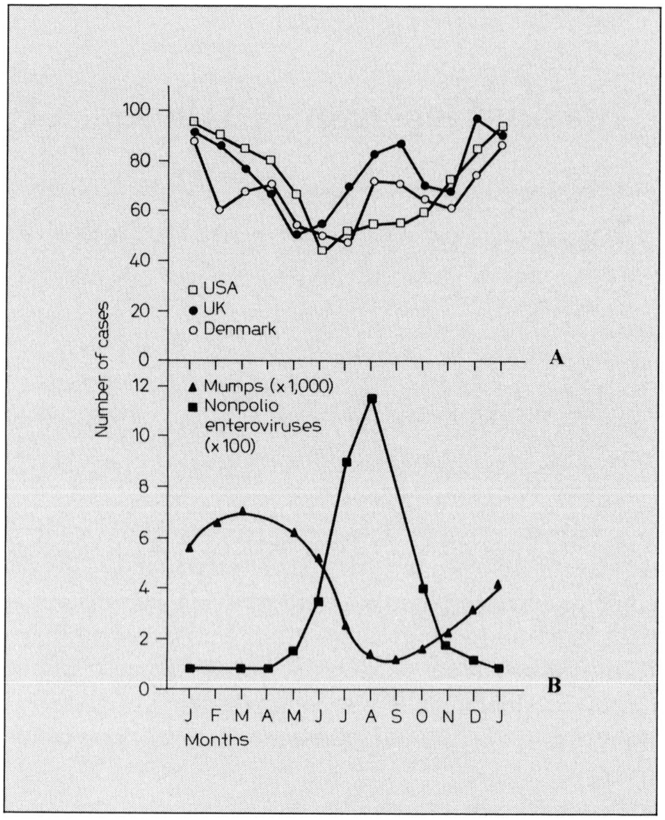

Fig. 1. **A** Seasonal incidence of new cases of insulin-dependent diabetes in USA, UK and Denmark. The incidence is higher during fall and winter. In the southern hemisphere this pattern is 6 months offset from this cycle. **B** Seasonal distribution of mumps and enteroviral infections in the northern hemisphere. These viruses are among the suspected diabetogenic agents. Adapted from ref. 6, 55, 56.

Viral Antibodies in IDDM

A number of studies comparing viral antibodies in diabetic and nondiabetic patients were stimulated by the early observation of Gamble et al. [6] who reported that higher mean antibody titers to Coxsackievirus B4 (CBV-4) were present in patients tested at the onset of acute diabetes than in patients with diabetes of longer duration or in normal controls [6]. These results were partially confirmed in a later study by the same group showing that this conclusion holds only in those cases with a relatively late onset of the disease (i.e., in age groups 10–19 and over 20 years). In fact, young patients aged 0–9 years had a lower prevalence of CBV-4 antibodies compared to age-matched controls. Investigations in Denmark and in the US confirmed this notion showing that early IDDM (i.e., before age 15) is associated with a low antibody response to CBV-3 and CBV-4 viruses [9]. An increased prevalence of antibodies to CBV-4 was also reported in Indian patients, but other studies from all over the world gave negative or equivocal results. Together with scattered reports, a recent multicenter study of Banatvala et al. [10, 11] seems to confirm the concept that in several cases recent CBV infections are associated with IDDM. Virus-specific IgM antibodies (i.e., a serologic sign of recent infection) were detected, in fact, in approximately one-third of the cases and were predominantly directed to CBV-4 and CBV-5.

Table I. Prevalence of viral antibodies in insulin-dependent diabetes of recent onset

Virus		Diabetic patients		Healthy controls	
family	species	% positive	total	% positive	total
Picorna	Coxsackie B-1	26.1	329	23.6	414
	Coxsackie B-2	46.3	289	44.9	394
	Coxsackie B-3	45.3	289	47.2	394
	Coxsackie B-4	62.8*	347	56.0	417
	Coxsackie B-5	36.1	329	41.0	414
	Coxsackie B-6	7.2	96	7.3	68
	Coxsackie B-group (IgM) (age group 0.5–15 years)	40.7*	221	22.7	431
	encephalomyocarditis	12.1	41	6.0	66
Paramyxo	mumps	66.7*	138	50.9	163
	measles	60.3*	156	40.6	155
Toga	rubella	76.5+	200	85.4	131
	VEE	10.4	86	7.1	98
Herpes	cytomegalovirus	41.7	67	32.0	25
Reo	reovirus-1	23.9+	96	56.7	104
	reovirus-2	51.0+	96	66.3	104
	reovirus-3	83.3+	96	98.0	104
Papova	BK	76.6	124	76.6	30

Cumulated data from various sources [9–12 and 57–64; Corallini, A., manuscript in preparation; Toniolo, A., manuscript in preparation].
* Significantly more prevalent in diabetics.
\+ Significantly less prevalent in diabetics.

Serologic investigations on the role of viruses other than CBVs have been rather limited in scope. For this reason, we collected data from published reports concerning the antibody response to several viruses potentially linked to human diabetes (table I).

It is apparent that, in general, antibodies to CBV-4 and specific IgM to the Coxsackie B virus group were detected more frequently in diabetics than in normal controls. The same conclusion can possibly apply also to cytomegalovirus and to mumps virus. In contrast, the antibody response to reovirus type 1 and 3 [12] and to the rubella virus appears significantly reduced in the patients studied so far. Reports from the US, Venezuela and Italy indicate that both the prevalence and the mean titers of antibodies to other agents such as encephalomyocarditis virus, Venezuelan encephalitis, measles and BK virus are not significantly different in patients and in controls.

Though different conclusions were drawn in individual reports, it appears that alterations of the antibody response to CBVs (particularly type B4), mumps, cytomegalovirus, rubella and reoviruses are present in a significant proportion of patients with IDDM, even though serum immunoglobulin levels at the onset of IDDM are approximately normal [12]. In contrast, the humoral response to other agents seems normal. Thus these studies suggest that certain viral infections are irrelevant to diabetogenesis. In general, an increased response to a given virus has been interpreted as if patients underwent infections with these agents at a higher than normal frequency. In contrast, when a lower than expected frequency of positives was found in diabetic patients, it was postulated that people developing diabetes early in life have some defects of the immune response to certain viruses. This interpretation seems reinforced by recent

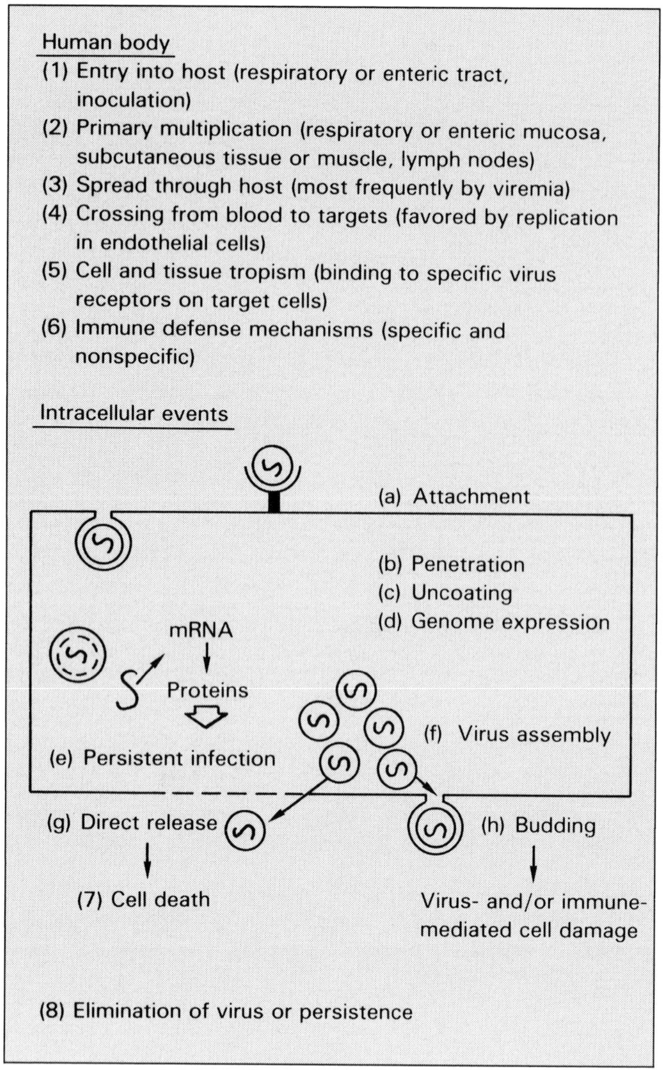

Fig. 2. Major pathogenetic mechanisms in virus-induced disease.

studies showing a defective cell-mediated immune response to mumps virus and to CBV-4 in HLA/DR3 individuals [13]. Thus, selective defects of the anti-infectious immune defenses might pose certain individuals at an increased risk of contracting diabetes.

It is not surprising, however, that no firm conclusions can be drawn from the serologic studies performed so far. These, in fact, have looked at common viruses to which approximately one-half of the population has been exposed at some time in life, and there are cases of diabetic patients lacking antibodies against most of the candidate viruses. Therefore, it seems likely that any of several viruses may act as a triggering agent of diabetes, but that the hypothetic etiologic agent(s) has still to be found.

Major Pathogenetic Mechanisms in Virus-Induced Disease

Viral pathogenesis is an intriguing multifactorial process, and our current understanding of the involved factors is still very incomplete [14]. The major pathogenetic steps are summarized in figure 2. Experimental studies on viral diabetes suggest that viruses can reach pancreatic islets mainly through the blood stream. In the islets of Langerhans, the afferent arterioles enter at discontinuities of the peripheral mantle of nonbeta cells, then break into capillaries that traverse the beta cell core and coalesce into collecting venules at the other side of the islets [15]. Capillaries of the islets have fenestred gaps in the endothelium, and in these spaces, two basement membranes separate endocrine cells from blood. The mechanism of transport of viruses across the endothelial cells and basement membrane is unknown, but it is known that the capillary blood flow in the islets is regulated by the innervation and the metabolic activity of endocrine cells. Thus, transient changes of blood flow and of capillary permeability might favor the penetration of viruses into islets. Once a virus has reached a tissue, its tropism is mediated by the interaction of specific viral polypeptides with specific cell receptors on the plasma membrane. Both these structures are under genetic control and are thus highly variable. This concept is of utmost relevance for the pathogenesis of viral diseases and allows one to envision how (1) variants of the same virus may exhibit different tropism, (2) the expression of cell receptors for viruses may vary among different individuals and different cell types in the same host and (3) the expression of receptors may vary in relation to the physiologic state of the cell. Factors other than receptors, however, may be important at the cellular level (i.e., specific enzymes required for virus replication, etc.). In addition, other factors of the host (such as the interferon system and the immune response to the infecting agent) exert a decisive influence on the outcome of viral infections.

In vitro and in vivo studies have clearly established that viruses can injure cells in at least four distinct ways: (1) The first is a lethal attack by toxic products of the viral genome or disruption of regulatory functions needed for cell survival. Thus, the virus itself directly destroys the cell. (2) The second way is indirect and occurs with cytopathic as well as noncytopathic viruses. The virus produces antigens foreign to the host or alters host antigens on the cell surface, thus the immune system indirectly kills such modified cells. Both these mechanisms yield similar results and have rather rapid pathologic consequences. (3) Virus infection triggers the production of autoantibodies that react with antigens of normal cells, thus also injuring cells that had not been infected previously. As a consequence, tissue injury is considerably delayed in respect of the infectious event. (4) Some variants of noncytopathic viruses cause persistent infections in vivo without altering the viability and the antigenicity of infected tissues. These viruses, however, may induce functional disorders in infected cells that are reflected in a reduced synthesis of hormonal products or of other 'luxury' functions. In this case, the disease is characterized by an insidious onset and by the lack of inflammatory changes in infected tissue.

In relating a particular disease with an infectious event, we are familiar with the relatively short incubation periods of most common viral diseases. In contrast, it should be borne in mind that animal and human studies have shown that the time between infection and the development of overt disease may range from only a few hours up to several decades.

The Pancreas as a Target for Viruses

Clinical and experimental observations indicate that pancreatic involvement occurs with a variety of virus infections. Due to the difficulty of clinical diagnosis, it is likely that mild forms of pancreatic damage are more common than is usually recognized. As shown in table II, multiple viruses have been associated with pancreatic disease and, in a number of cases, it has been possible to establish the main target cell for each agent. Although target tissues may vary in different animal species, it appears that most pancreatotropic viruses replicate in acinar cells; in contrast, ductal epithelial cells seems to be infected more rarely, e.g. by reoviruses and cytomegalovirus.

Endocrine cells appear quite resistant to infection under natural conditions, and knowledge of their involvement mostly derives from animal models as well as from the study of rare human cases. It is noteworthy that islet cells are usually spared by infection even in the course of massive virus replication in exocrine tissue as seen, for instance in Coxsackie B virus infections (fig. 3A–C). Undoubtely, this reflects the existence of some unknown mechanisms which protect islets from viral invasion. Thus involvement of islet cells is due predominantly to infection with particular (betatropic) variants of common viruses usually sparing the acinar tissue (fig. 3D), or it occurs in connection with overwhelming viral infections.

Table II. The pancreas as a target for viruses

Virus	Host	Main target cell		
		acinar	ductal	endocrine
Coxsackie group-B	human mouse	+	–	+
Foot-and-mouth disease	cattle	+	–	+
Encephalomyocarditis	mouse hamster guinea pig marmoset	+	–	+
Reovirus	mouse	±	+	+
Mumps	human	+	–	±
Varicella-zoster	human	+	–	+
Cytomegalovirus	human mouse	+	+	+
Venezuelan encephalitis	hamster	+	–	+
Retrovirus	chick mouse	+	±	+
Murine hepatitis	mouse	+	–	–
Rubella (CRS)	human hamster	?	?	±
Lymphocytic choriomeningitis	mouse	?	?	±
Epstein-Barr	human	?	?	?

The mechanism of pancreatic damage consequent to virus infection is incompletely understood, but it seems that the initial step in the process is the focal infection of the acinar tissue followed by cell necrosis and release of zymogen enzymes into the tissue. In contrast, other agents such as the rubella virus, apparently fail to destroy the acinar tissue and induce only interstitial pancreatitis.

As shown by experimental studies, the pancreas may represent also a target for the replication of viruses which fail to destroy target cells and to induce inflammatory changes. Among these are viruses responsible for chronic asymptomatic infections such as endogenous or exogenous retroviruses [16] and lymphocytic choriomeningitis virus [17]. The role of these agents in pancreatic disease is presently unknown, but they are suspected as a possible cause of functional alterations at the cellular level.

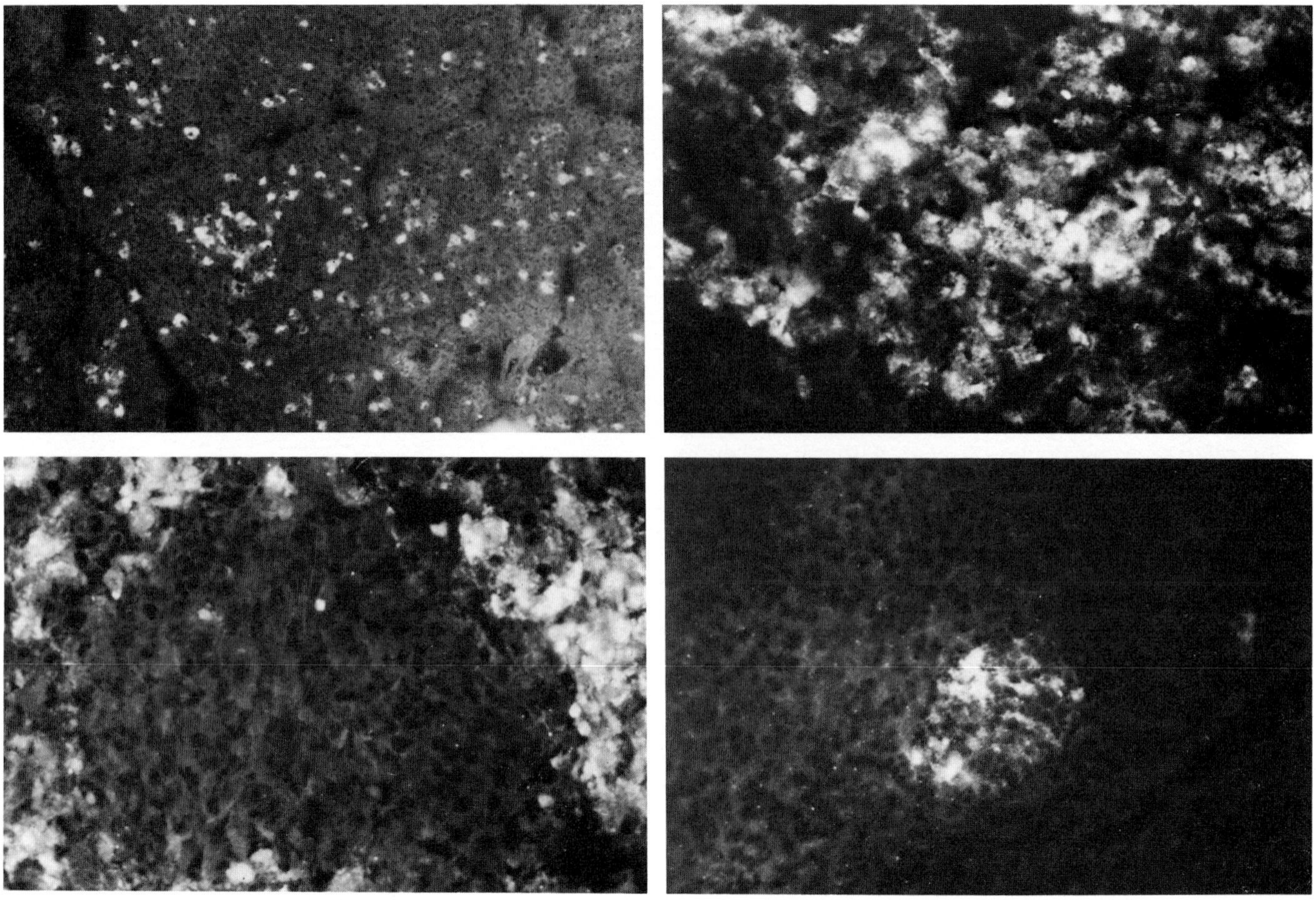

Fig. 3. Progression of pancreatitis induced by a common strain of Coxsackievirus B-3 in mice. Viral antigens were detected by immunofluorescence with antiviral antibody 18 h (**A**) or 72 h (**B, C**) after infection. The pancreatic islet seen in **C** is completely spared by infection in spite of the massive involvement of exocrine tissue. **D** Selective infection of islet cells by Coxsackievirus B-5. This strain was made betatropic by repeated passage in mouse beta cell cultures. It is evident that this virus has virtually lost its original tropism for the acinar tissue.

Virus-Induced Diabetes in Experimental Animals

Further evidence for the possibility of a viral etiology of certain forms of IDDM comes from animal studies. Since many excellent reviews on this topic have already been published [5–7, 18–21], we will here summarize the major conclusions of these studies. (1) Acute beta cell damage, insulitis, hypoinsulinemia and hyperglycemia may follow the infection of mice with highly lytic viruses, such as encephalomyocarditis (EMC) virus [22] and group B Coxsackieviruses [23, 24]. (2) Only selected 'betatropic' variants of these viruses can infect islet cells inducing diabetes [25]. In nature these agents occur as mixtures of different variants, some of which can infect beta cells. (3) EMC-induced diabetes is followed by long-term complications similar to those observed in human diabetes [26]. (4) In at least some cases, genetic factors control the susceptibility of mice to viral diabetogenesis; in contrast to human IDDM, however, the responsible genes are not linked to the major histocompatibility complex of the mouse. (5) Reovirus infection of newborn mice can result not only in diabetes, but also in the development of an autoimmune polyendocrine disease [27]. This disease is partially mediated by the production of autoantibodies to pancreatic islets, anterior pituitary and thyroid. Autoantibodies to insulin, growth hormone and thyroglobulin have also been detected. (6) Reovirus-induced diabetes can be prevented by immunosuppression [28]. (7) The exposure of mice to a series of subsequent insults from different viruses or from viruses and chemicals may result in a critical depletion of beta cells and in the development of hyperglycemia [29, 30]. (8) Persistent infections with certain nonlytic viruses (lymphocytic choriomeningitis virus and Venezuelan encephalitis virus) can produce a long-term reduction of insulin secretion and/or release without obvious pathologic changes of islets [17, 31].

For unknown reasons, strains of these candidate diabetogenic viruses, which are disseminated in the human population, are predominantly tropic for organs other than the endocrine pancreas. The existence of diabetogenic variants, however, is indirectly proved by the rare documented cases of virus-induced IDDM in humans as well as by the relatively frequent finding of insulitis and/or damage of pancreatic islets in patients dying of fatal viral infections. In addition, these studies in mice point to the possibility that a variety of interactions can occur among environmental agents at the beta cell level and that many different insults, occurring together or sequentially, may set the stage for the development of diabetes.

Virus-Induced Diabetes in Humans

Virus Infection of Human Beta Cells in vitro

Since it is difficult to ascertain if human beta cells are susceptible to viral infections in vivo, an in vitro system has been developed to determine which viruses are capable of infecting human beta cells in culture. Due to the difficulty of obtaining large quantities of functionally active beta cells, these studies have been rather limited in scope. Since these cultures are not composed of beta cells alone, a double-label immunofluorescent antibody technique has always been used to show unequivocally that it was the beta cell, and not contaminating nonbeta cells, that became infected.

By this method, the group of *Notkins* [32] showed that beta cells from seven human donors were permissive for the replication of mumps virus. This agent caused direct lysis of most beta cells in about 6 days, but also infected a sizeable proportion of nonbeta cells. In a series of similar experiments, *Yoon* et al. [33, 34] showed that also CBV-3, CBV-4, and selected strains of reo-3 cause rapid beta cell lysis accompanied by a remarkable decrease of intracellular immunoreactive insulin. In contrast, reo-3 strains which had not been passaged in beta cell cultures replicated only in a small percentage of beta cells, without altering the insulin content of cultured cells. It has also been shown that BK virus (a Papovavirus which may cause insulinoma in hamsters and intrauterine infection in humans) may infect and destroy human beta cells in vitro.

In most cases, human donors were not HLA typed, thus precluding any conclusion with regard to the influence of the genetic make-up of the host on virus susceptibility. Although it is known that virus susceptibility in vitro does not reflect necessarily the situation in vivo, further studies in this direction may help to identify naturally occurring betatropic viruses.

Postmortem Studies: Virus Capable of Infecting Pancreatic Islets in vivo

The finding that many viruses which are highly disseminated in humans may induce diabetes in experimental animals and may infect human beta cells in vitro raises the questions of whether and how frequently viral infections of human islet cells occur in vivo.

Theoretically, this problem should be approached by looking for histopathologic damage of pancreatic islets during the course of common virus infections. Since pancreatic biopsies cannot be obtained from patients, the only available information has been obtained from histopathologic studies of the rare patients dying of severe viral infections. Thus, in interpreting these data it should be borne in mind that the following findings refer to rather uncommon clinical cases. *Jenson* et al. [35], examining the pancreas of 250 children with fatal infections caused by at least 14 different viruses, found insular pathology in 28 cases. Other surveys have demonstrated insular changes in 15 of 85 cases of neonatal Coxsackie B virus infections, and cytopathology of the islets has also been reported in cases of disseminated infections due to cytomegalovirus, mumps, varicella-zoster and rubella virus [36–38]. Thus, damage of pancreatic islets has been found in at least 13% of fatal viral infections. In these studies the vast majority of pathologic changes was found in neonates, and in most cases islet cells other than beta cells were clearly involved. In cases due to lytic agents such as CBVs, some islet cells appeared to have undergone lysis and many others had dense pyknotic nuclei; most islets were mildly to moderately degranulated of insulin, and mononuclear cell infiltrates were present in 3–30% of islets. Islet cell involvement seems relatively frequent in cases of disseminated varicella-zoster infections. In this case, the infection of islets is focal and involves also adjacent acinar cells. The agent most frequently responsible for islet cells infection is, perhaps, cytomegalovirus. In fact, over 30 cases of islet cell damage due to this agent have been reported in the literature

[36]. Although most of these reports refer to congenital or neonatal infections, it appears that cytomegalovirus can also infect the islets of adult subjects. In this connection, it is noteworthy that at least one such case has been found in an adult male with AIDS [39]. Cytomegalovirus-infected cells are easily recognized by the large intranuclear inclusions which are found, usually but not always, in cells at the periphery on the islets. In addition to beta cells, other cell types are infected, and the virus appears to cause a mild to moderate loss of insulin granules. Perhaps due to the immunosuppressive activity of this agent, insulitis is a rare finding in these patients. Though the development of diabetes is a rather frequent sequela of the congenital rubella syndrome, histologic evidence for viral cytophatology and insulitis has been provided on rare occasions. In fact, only 2 cases with islet damage and mild insulitis have been described so far [40].

In a great porportion of the above cases, pathological changes of the islets were more prominent than those in the surrounding acinar tissue, suggesting that a subpopulation of the virus pool may have had a specific tropism for islet cells. Thus, these studies do provide further in vivo support for the observation that, under certain circumstances, viruses can infect and damage human beta cells.

Clinical Cases

The best way to establish a direct link between viral infections and human diabetes is, obviously, the recovery of viruses from diabetic patients and the demonstration that the isolated agents are capable of causing diabetes in experimental hosts.

So far, this goal has been achieved in only two cases. The first is that of a 10-year-old boy who developed diabetic ketoacidosis within 3 days after the onset of a flu-like illness. Despite intensive therapy, his conditions deteriorated and he died 7 days later. At autopsy, insulitis and necrosis of beta cells were observed. *Yoon* et al. [41] were able to isolate a variant of CBV-4 from the pancreas. Studies of the patient's serum revealed a rise in the titer of neutralizing antibody to this isolate from less than 4 on the second hospital day, to 32 on the day of death. In addition, viral antigens were detected by immunofluorescence in various organs of the child. This provided clear evidence that at the time of death CBV-4 was causing a systemic infection, and that the isolated virus was not an inadvertent contaminant from the laboratory. To prove that this agent was truly related to the child's diabetes, several inbred strains of mice were inoculated with the CBV-4 isolate. Susceptible mice developed acute diabetes, while mice of resistant strains did not. Moreover, examination of the pancreas from diabetic mice revealed acute insulitis, destruction of beta cells, and the presence of viral antigens in the islets of Langerhans. All these data led to the conclusion that the patient's diabetes was virus-induced.

The second case is that of a 16-month-old girl who was hospitalized for thrombocytopenic purpura appearing after 1 week of fever. Laboratory evidence of diabetes was present from days 13 to 25, then a remission ensued, but 2 months later the child developed overt IDDM [42]. On the 8th day after the onset of fever, CBV-5 was isolated from the stools. Antibody titers to this agent rose from less than 10 to 640, showing that in the period preceding the onset of diabetes the baby had been infected by CBV-5. When this isolate was inoculated into various strains of inbred mice, glucose intolerance was produced in those strains which are susceptible to the diabetogenic effects of encephalomyocarditis virus. Since the common strains of CBV-5 do not produce diabetes in mice, it was concluded that this child had been infected by a betatropic variant of this virus. The high-risk genetic markers DR3 and BfF1 were present in this patient and, at the time of hospitalization, she had elevated titers of islet cells antibodies. Thus it appears that in this case CBV-5 infection contributed with genetic and immunologic factors to the production of diabetes.

In other cases the proof that the isolated agents could induce diabetes in experimental animals has not been provided. Nevertheless, in the following cases a virus was identified and its relation to the disease was established by histopathologic findings. One was a 5-year-old girl who developed myocarditis and acute diabetes 7 days after open-heart surgery [43]. She died in diabetic ketoacidosis. At autopsy degeneration and necrosis of islet cells and an associated insulitis were seen in the pancreas. CBV-4 antigens were found in the islets by immunofluorescence, and high levels of antibody to this virus were found in the serum. Thus it appeared that the development of IDDM in this girl was the direct consequence of acute CBV-4 infection.

One case of diabetes due to CBV-1 infection occurred in a newborn twin who acquired the virus from the mother a few days before birth [38]. Immediately after birth his conditions deteriorated and he developed thrombocytopenia and myocardiopathy. On day 12 blood glucose rose to over 500 mg/dl, and he died 4 days later. At necropsy, pancreatic lesions consisted of insulitis with islet cell degeneration, and CBV-1 was recovered from the pancreas. It is interesting to notice that his twin brother, though developing a severe disease due to the same strain of CBV-1, did not become diabetic and could be discharged from the hospital 25 days after birth. Thus it appears that, even in humans, infection with a diabetogenic virus does not result always in the development of diabetes.

An 11-year-old boy, who was under therapy with corticosteroids for idiopathic thrombocytopenia, died 4 days after developing a disseminated infection and concomitant diabetes. Typical cytomegalovirus inclusions, without insulitits, were found in the islets of Langerhans [35]. There were normal numbers of beta cells which appeared, however, to be only partially granulated.

Another case was that of a 14-month-old boy with well-documented congenital rubella syndrome (CRS) [40]. He died 5 days after developing diabetes. Insulin-containing beta cells could not be detected. A subacute insulitis was observed, but most islets were partially hyalinized, indicating prior damage.

Other cases of acute-onset IDDM have been associated with various viral infections on less solid grounds. So far, over 15 additional cases have been reported: 1 was attributed to CBV-1, 1 to CBV-2, 2 to CBV-5, 3 to mumps virus, 5 to Epstein-Barr virus (the etiologic agent of infectious mononucleosis) and some others to the rubella virus [38, 44–46].

It is difficult to establish whether in these cases the reported viral agents were directly responsible for the development of IDDM or whether they acted merely as triggering factors superimposed on an ongoing diabetogenic process. Those cases which have been reported during the neonatal period, however, represent undoubtely a direct consequence of the viral attack. Although many questions remain, these studies support the contention that at least some cases of IDDM have a viral etiology.

Diabetes and the Congenital Rubella Syndrome: A Possible Link between Viruses and Genetic Factors in Causing Autoimmunity and Diabetes.

The most convincing evidence that a persistent virus infection may cause IDDM derives from studies of patients with CRS. It has been shown that after intrauterine infection the rubella virus can be isolated from patients for over 20 years and that, among other organs, it can produce persistent infection of the pancreas. Prospective studies from Australia, the US and other countries have established that the prevalence of diabetes among CRS patients is extraordinarily high (5–20%) and that a latent period of many years is required for the disease to develop [47, 48]. So far, over 60 cases of diabetes have been reported worldwide in CRS patients and the mean age of onset was approximately 13 years (range 1–30). The finding that the disease is highly prevalent and has a long latent period in these subjects makes CRS patients an ideal group for the study of the pathogenetic events preceding diabetes. Accordingly, it has been observed that cytoplasmic and/or surface islet cell antibodies are found in over 20% of the total CRS population and in more than 70% of those who will develop diabetes [49]. In addition, many CRS patients have thyroid autoantibodies, showing that persistent infection with this agent can stimulate endocrine autoimmunity against several organs. *Rubinstein* et al. [48] have shown that only those CRS subjects having the high-risk genetic markers (DR3 and/or DR4) become diabetic, and that the disease develops in virtually all these individuals. In contrast, as in other cases of IDDM, the DR2 genotype affords protection. Thus it appears that this severe intrauterine infection can push the penetrance of the common susceptibility genotype towards 100%. How this virus induces diabetes is unknown, but this model indicates that a persistent viral insult, together with a permissive genotype, can trigger an autoimmune response leading to beta cell failure (fig. 4).

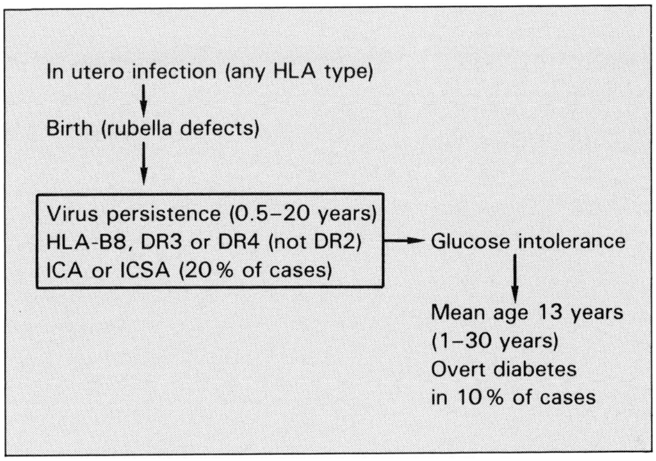

Fig. 4. Congenital rubella syndrome: the cooperation of viral, genetic, and immunologic factors in causing diabetes.

Besides rubella virus, a number of other betatropic viruses have the potential to infect the fetus without necessarily causing immediate pathological effects: among them cytomegalovirus, mumps and BK virus. Therefore, the question arises whether exposure to these agents in utero does predispose to diabetes.

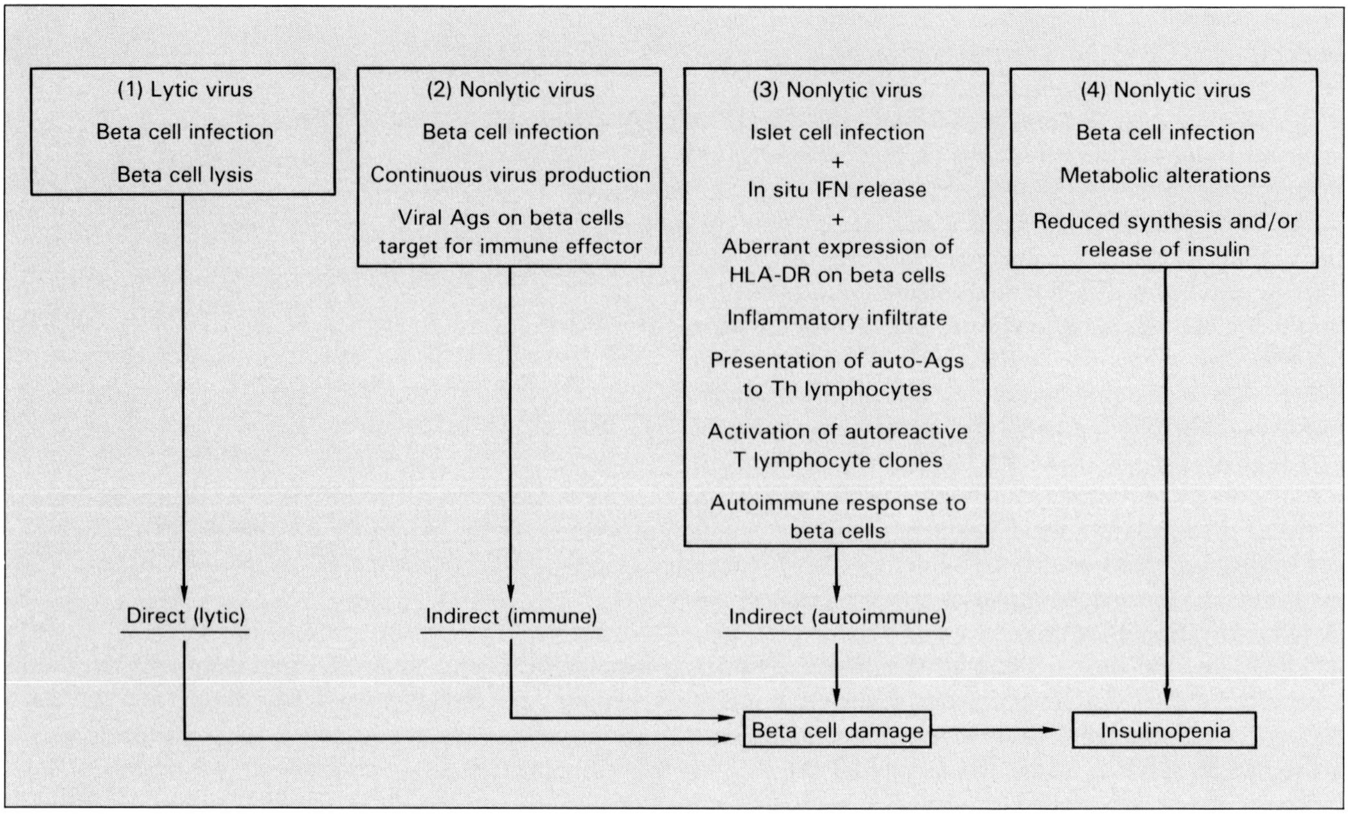

Fig. 5. Pathogenesis of virus-induced diabetes. Models requiring virus infection of beta cells.

Possible Mechanisms Leading from Virus Infection to the Production of Diabetes in Humans

Experimental studies on virus-induced diabetes, together with the few reported human cases of viral etiology, indicate that certain viruses can damage pancreatic beta cells. Based on our current views of viral pathogenesis [14] it is possible to envision four major pathways leading from viral infection of islet cells to the development of the disease (fig. 5):

(1) The first possibility is that of a lytic virus tropic for beta cells. The intracellular replication of this agent directly kills the cell, and diabetes ensues a few days or a few weeks within the onset of a systemic infection. In animals a similar process is caused by EMC virus, foot-and-mouth disease virus and CBVs. In humans, it may be associated with the few described cases of CBV-induced diabetes which were usually lethal.

(2) The second mechanism may be triggered by a persistent infection of beta cells with a nonlytic or mildly lytic agent. In this case, beta cell failure would be promoted by an immune attack against viral antigens expressed on the surface of beta cells. Thus the immune system indirectly kills virus-replicating cells. This process is notably slower than the first one since it requires the triggering of an antiviral immune response as well as the penetration of immune effectors into the islets. Albeit this mechanism is activated in the course of most viral infections, it may be of particular relevance to the pathogenesis of those forms of human diabetes due to slow-replicating agents such as rubella or cytomegalovirus.

(3) It is widely accepted that viruses can induce autoimmunity, but the precise mechanisms are unknown. The third model thus refers to a proposed pathway leading from a local insult to organ-specific autoimmunity [50]. It has been observed that HLA class II antigens are highly expressed in certain endocrine tissues from patients with a variety of autoimmune endocrine diseases. Since the expression of these molecules is normally restricted to antigen-presenting cells, B lymphocytes, activated T lymphocytes, thymic epithelium and to certain endothelial cells, the finding of these antigens on epithelial cells is

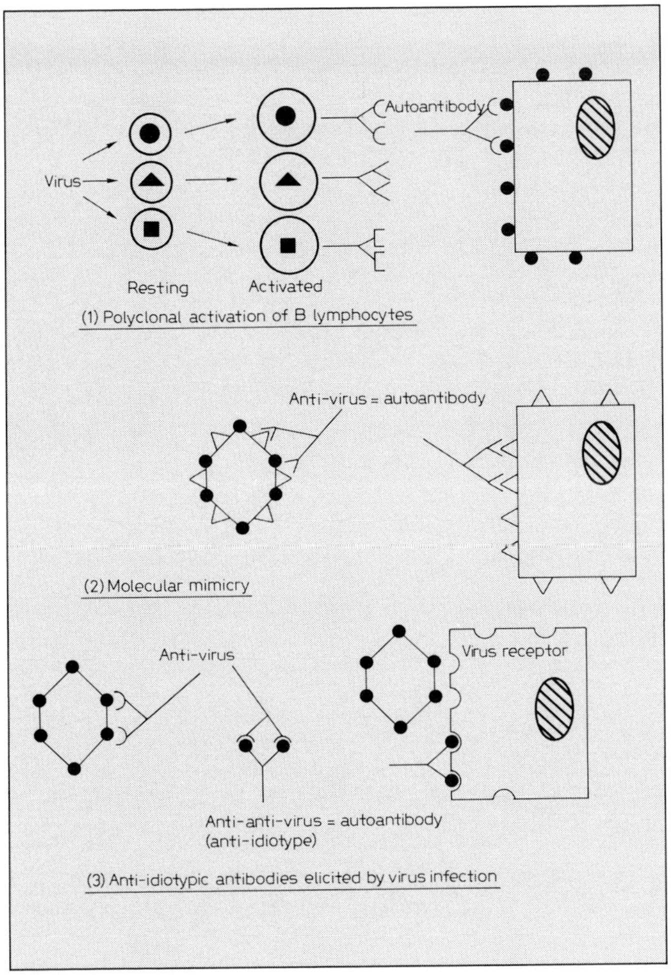

Fig. 6. Pathogenesis of virus-induced diabetes. Models not requiring virus infection of beta cells.

Table III. Pancreatic autoantibodies from cultures of EBV-infected human B lymphocytes from normal subjects

Donor	Positive cultures, %			
	islet cells	acinar tissue	ducts and ductules	smooth muscle
1	25	27	62	62
2	24	24	53	41

10^4 purified B lymphocytes from normal individuals were infected in vitro with EBV. Three weeks later, culture supernatants were tested for IgM autoantibodies to frozen sections of human pancreas by avidin-biotin immunoperoxidase.

considered an 'aberrant expression' of the HLA-D region products. If other cells which are not designed for antigen processing and/or presentation do express HLA-D molecules, these cells may become antigen-presenting cells upon interaction with lymphocytes [51], since the physiologic role of these molecules is to allow the interaction of macrophages with lymphocytes during antigen presentation. It has been shown that in vitro endocrine cells do express DR molecules if exposed to physiological concentrations of interferon (IFN). In the islets of Langerhans in vivo, this sequence of events might be triggered by the local production of IFN in response to a viral infection. Under these conditions, beta cells would have the opportunity of presenting autoantigens to autoreactive T helper lymphocytes. Thus an autoimmune response to beta cells would be triggered.

Since the IFN response is not virus-specific, any insulotropic virus could theoretically initiate this sequence. Though hypothetical, this mechanism would explain our present incapacity to associate specific causal viruses with diabetes and would justify the long prediabetic period observed in IDDM. In fact, the infection might occur months to years before the onset of overt disease and initiate a slow autoimmune damage.

(4) The fourth mechanism refers to viruses producing silent infections of beta cells. Such agents have never been detected in the human pancreas. In mice, however, a long-term reduction of insulin synthesis or release in the absence of any obvious damage to beta cells has been observed after persistent infection with LCM or VEE [17, 31]. This effect is presumably due to the subversion of the insulin biosynthetic machinery by the virus replicative cycle. Thus, these agents produce an insulinopenic syndrome mimicking certain forms of type-II diabetes.

Experiment work in viral immunology suggests that viruses might cause an autoimmune response to pancreatic islets by mechanisms other than islet cell infection [52] (fig. 6):

(1) One possibility is that the virus triggers autoimmunity by acting on the immunoregulatory system. One of the best examples comes from studies with Epstein-Barr virus (EBV) [53]. EBV is a human virus that selectively infects B lymphocytes and causes infectious mononucleosis. In vitro, this agent transforms resting B lymphocytes into lymphoblastoid cell lines with indefinite life span that proliferate and secrete immunoglobulins of different specificities.

As shown in table III, cultures of B lymphocytes from normal donors infected in vitro with EBV produce autoantibodies against pancreatic antigens, including islet

A B C D

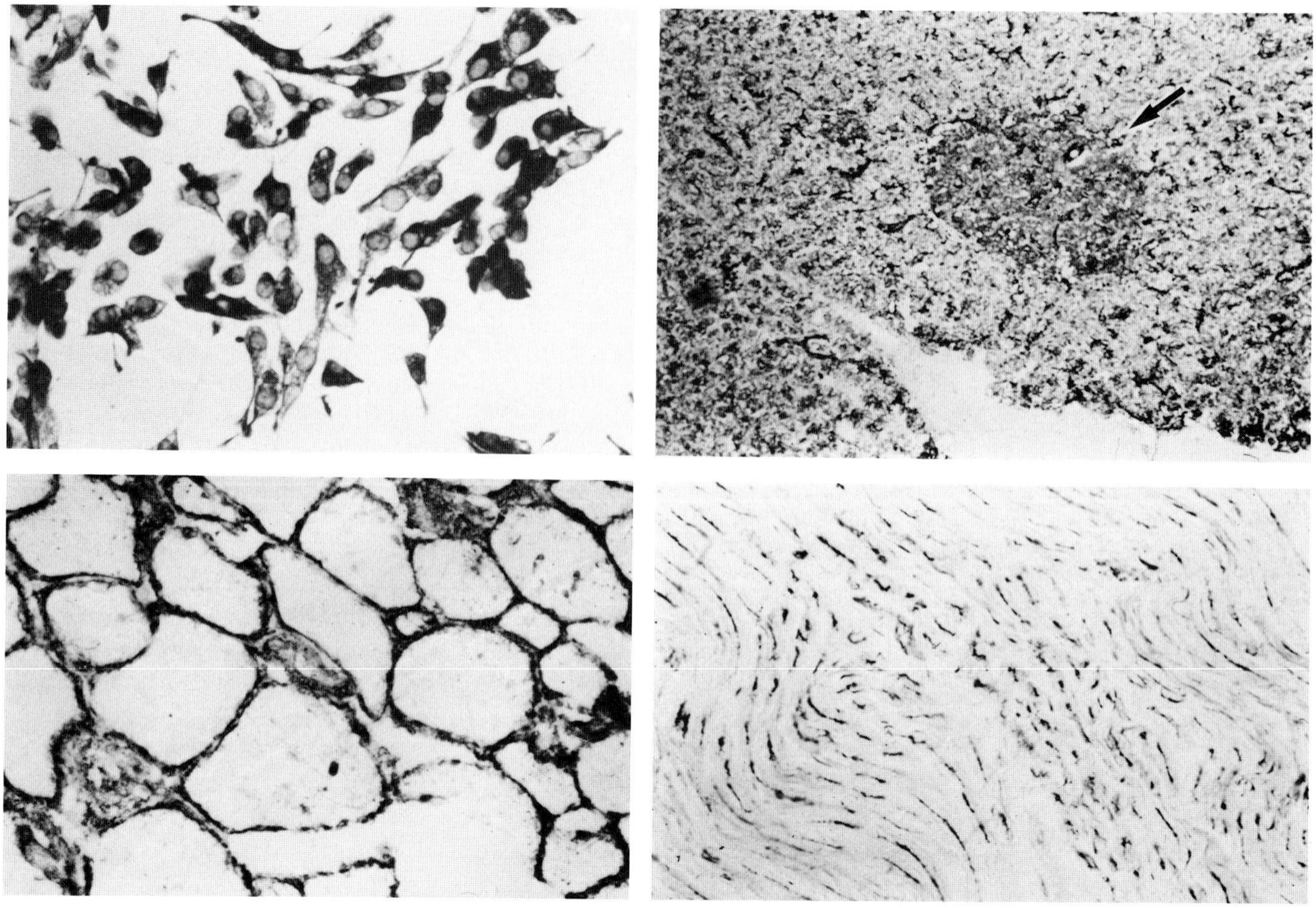

Fig. 7. Reactivity of a human monoclonal IgM autoantibody produced by EBV-transformed B lymphocytes. This antibody, selected for reactivity to rat insulinoma cells (**A**), also binds to human pancreatic islets (**B**), thyroid acinar cells (**C**) and axons of peripheral nerve (**D**). Antibodies of this type have been termed 'multiple-organ-reactive'. Indirect staining of unfixed frozen sections with avidin-biotin immunoperoxidase.

cells. This is regarded as a consequence of virus-induced polyclonal B cell activation, during which resting B lymphocyte clones are triggered to express their immunoglobulin repertoire, including autoantibodies. This experimental evidence makes it clear that a virus can induce the production of autoantibodies through its lymphoproliferative effect without infecting the target cells to which the autoantibodies are directed.

Some of the anti-islet autoantibodies produced by EBV-infected B lymphocytes have been cloned and studied in detail, and most of them have been found to react with antigens in multiple organs. One example of these multiple-organ-reactive autoantibodies is given in figure 7. The demonstration of polyreactivity of many monoclonal autoantibodies is of particular interest, since autoantibodies that react with a variety of organs (i.e., thyroid, gastric mucosa, adrenals, anterior pituitary, lymphocytes) are often found in the serum of IDDM patients, and the nature of this multiple-organ autoreactivity of serum has never been fully explained.

In vivo, EBV is thought to similarly induce lymphoproliferation and autoantibody production, but this phenomenon is usually transient because infected B lymphocytes are killed by cytotoxic T lymphocytes. Thus, persistent autoantibody production might occur in individuals with immunoregulatory defects.

(2) Another possibility is that of 'molecular mimicry'. The idea is that antibodies raised against certain viral antigens may cross-react with normal host cell antigens. Monoclonal antibodies to viruses are now beginning to

substantiate this hypothesis. For instance, cross-reactivity has been observed between certain viral antigens and intermediate filaments, thymic epithelium, pituitary cells and islet cells. Thus, infection with agents having structural similarities with islet cell constituents might result in the production of autoimmune diabetes.

(3) A third mechanism by which a virus could trigger an autoimmune response is by eliciting anti-idiotypic antibodies. Anti-idiotypic antibodies are viewed as regulatory immunoglobulins directed to the idiotype of a particular antibody. As a consequence, these molecules not only react with the variabile site of the antiviral antibody, but also are structurally analogous to the eliciting antigen. If this antigen is the viral structure which binds to the viral receptors on host cells, the anti-idiotype antibody also recognizes the viral receptor and binds to the cell membrane. Only a few examples of this type have been found so far, but this is an appealing mechanism since it would lead to the production of potentially hazardous surface autoantibodies.

Conclusions

The studies on viral diabetes demonstrate that several different viruses can cause the disease or contribute to pathogenesis. In humans, however, only a few cases of virus-induced diabetes have been described so far. The fact that autoimmune phenomena together with alterations of lymphocyte subsets precede the clinical onset of the disease by months or years makes one wonder if a persistent infection with a slow virus occurred well before overt diabetes. If this were the case, it is possible that newer virological techniques will allow the isolation of this unknown agent opening the road to prevention. On the other hand, it appears equally possible that most cases of IDDM derive primarily from 'spontaneous' autoimmunity, and that viruses or other environmental factors act merely as triggering agents. In this case, preventive measures would be much more difficult.

The solution of this pathogenetic puzzle would be facilitated by the correct understanding of the relationships between HLA type, autoimmunity and viral infections. Nevertheless, even if we actually do not know why people carrying certain genetic markers are prone to diabetes or to other autoimmune diseases, our comprehension of several chronic 'idiopathic' diseases has advanced very fast in the last years [54]. Various forms of chronic hepatitis, subacute sclerosing panencephalitis, kuru, multiple sclerosis, the acquired immunodeficiency syndrome and some forms of neoplasia have been attributed to conventional or to unconventional viruses. To make this issue even more complex, it is clear that some of these diseases represent unusual responses of the host to an infectious agent. If this were also true for IDDM, the identification of the putative etiologic agent(s) will require enormous efforts. Undoubtedly this search will join together investigators from various disciplines and will further progress in many fields of endocrinology.

Acknowledgements

We thank Dr. *A.L. Notkins* for introducing us to this area of research and for his continuous encouragement and support. We are also grateful to Drs. *J.W. Yoon, A.B. Jenson, T. Onodera, M.J. Dobersen, G.F. Bottazzo, C. Betterle, B. Prabhakar, F.E. Taub, I. Manocchio, G. Federspil, S. Mariotti* and *A. Corallini* for illuminating discussions and collaboration. This work was supported by the Italian Ministry of Education (funds 40% and 60%), and by Novo Farmaceutici Italia through the courtesy of Dr. *M. Iavicoli.*

References

1 Irvine, W.J.: Classification of diabetes mellitus; in Andreani, Di Mario, Federlin, Heding, Immunology in diabetes, pp. 283–294 (Kimpton, London 1984).

2 Gorsuch, A.N.; Spencer, K.M.; Lister, J.; McNally, J.M.; Dean, B.M.; Bottazzo, G.F.; Cudworth, A.G.: Evidence for a long prediabetic period in type I (insulin-dependent) diabetes mellitus. Lancet *ii:* 1363–1365 (1981).

3 Pyke, D.A.: Diabetes: the genetic connections. Diabetologia *17:* 333–343 (1979).

4 Like, A.A.; Rossini, A.A.: Streptozotocin-induced pancreatic insulitis: new model of diabetes mellitus. Science *193:* 415–417 (1976).

5 Craighead, J.E.: The role of viruses in the pathogenesis of pancreatic disease and diabetes mellitus. Prog. med. Virol., vol. 19, pp. 161–214 (Karger, Basel 1975).

6 Gamble, D.R.: The epidemiology of insulin-dependent diabetes with particular reference to the relationship of virus infection to its etiology. Epidemiol. Rev. *2:* 49–70 (1980).

7 Rayfield, E.J.; Seto, Y.: Viruses; in Brownlee, Handbook of diabetes mellitus, vol. 1, pp. 95–120 (Garland, New York 1981).

8 Gamble, D.R.: Relation of antecedent illness to development of diabetes in children. Br. med. J. *ii:* 99–101 (1980).

9 Palmer, J.P.; Cooney, M.K.; Ward, R.M.; Hansen, J.A.; Brodsky, J.B.; Ray, C.G.; Crossley, J.R.; Asplin, C.M.; Williams, R.M.: Reduced Coxsackie antibody titers in type I (insulin-dependent) diabetic patients presenting during an outbreak of Coxsackie B3 and B4 infection. Diabetologia *22:* 426–429 (1982).

10 Banatvala, J.E.; Bryant, J.; Schernthaner, G.; Borkenstein, M,; Schober, E.; Brown, D.; De Silva, L.M.; Menser, M.A.; Silink, M..: Coxsackie B, mumps, rubella, and cytomegalovirus specific IgM responses in patients with juvenile-onset insulin-dependent diabetes mellitus in Britain, Austria, and Australia. Lancet *i:* 1409–1412 (1985).

11 Gamble, D.R.; Cumming, H.: Coxsackie B virus and juvenile-onset insulin-dependent diabetes. Lancet *ii:* 455–456 (1985).
12 Toniolo, A.; Conaldi, P.G.; Garzelli, C.; Benedettini, G.; Federico, G.; Saggese, G.; Vettor, R.; Federspil, G.: Role of antecedent mumps and reovirus infections on the development of type I (insulin-dependent) diabetes. Eur. J. Epidemiol. *1:* 172–179 (1985).
13 Bruserud, O.; Jervell, J.; Thorsby, E.: HLA-DR3 and -DR4 control T-lymphocyte responses to mumps and Coxsackie B4 virus: studies on patients with type 1 (insulin-dependent) diabetes and healthy subjects. Diabetologia *28:* 420–426 (1985).
14 Mims, C.A.; White, D.O.: Viral pathogenesis and immunology, pp. 1–398 (Blackwell, Oxford 1984).
15 Bonner-Weir, S.; Orci, L.: New perspectives on the microvasculature of the islets of Langerhans in the rat. Diabetes *31:* 883–889 (1982).
16 Leiter, E.H.: Type C retrovirus production by pancreatic beta cells. Association with accelerated pathogenesis in C3H-db/db ('diabetes') mice. Am. J. Path. *119:* 22–32 (1985).
17 Oldstone, M.B.A.; Southern, P.; Rodriguez, M.; Lampert, P.: Virus persists in beta cells of islets of Langerhans and is associated with chemical manifestations of diabetes. Science *224:* 1440–1443 (1984).
18 Craighead, J.E.: Viral diabetes mellitus in man and experimental animals. Am. J. Med. *70:* 127–135 (1981).
19 Notkins, A.L.: Virus-induced diabetes mellitus. Brief review. Archs Virol. *54:* 1–17 (1977).
20 Notkins, A.L.: The causes of diabetes. Scient. Am. *241:* 62–73 (1979).
21 Toniolo, A.; Onodera, T.: Viruses and diabetes; in Andreani, Di Mario, Federlin, Heding, Immunology in diabetes, pp. 71–93 (Kimpton, London 1984).
22 Yoon, J.W.; Onodera, T.; Notkins, A.L.: Virus-induced diabetes mellitus. VIII. Passage of encephalomyocarditis virus and severity of diabetes in susceptible and resistant strains of mice. J. gen. Virol. *37:* 225–232 (1977).
23 Yoon, J.W.; Onodera, T.; Notkins, A.L.: Virus-induced diabetes mellitus. XV. Beta cell damage and insulin-dependent hyperglycemia in mice infected with Coxsackievirus B4. J. exp. Med. *148:* 1068–1080 (1978).
24 Toniolo, A.; Onodera, T.; Jordan, G.; Yoon, J.W.; Notkins, A.L.: Virus-induced diabetes mellitus: glucose abnormalities produced in mice by the six members of the Coxsackie B virus group. Diabetes *31:* 496–499 (1982).
25 Yoon, J.W.; McClintock, P.R.; Onodera, T.; Notkins, A.L.: Virus-induced diabetes mellitus. XVIII. Inhibition by a non-diabetogenic variant of encephalomyocarditis virus. J. exp. Med. *152:* 878–892 (1980).
26 Yoon, J.W.; Rodrigues, M.M.; Currier, C.; Notkins, A.L.: Long-term complications of virus-induced diabetes mellitus in mice. Nature *296:* 566–569 (1982).
27 Onodera, T.; Toniolo, A.; Ray, U.R.; Jenson, A.B.; Knazek, A.; Notkins, A.L.: Virus-induced diabetes mellitus. XX. Polyendocrinopathy and autoimmunity. J. exp. Med. *153:* 1457–1473 (1981).
28 Onodera, T.; Ray, U.R.; Melez, K.A.; Suzuki, H.; Toniolo, A.; Notkins, A.L.: Virus-induced diabetes mellitus: autoimmunity and polyendocrine disease prevented by immunosuppression. Nature *297:* 66–68 (1982).
29 Toniolo, A.; Onodera, T.; Yoon, J.W.; Notkins, A.L.: Induction of diabetes by cumulative environmental insults from viruses and chemicals. Nature *288:* 383–385 (1980).
30 Onodera, T.; Suzuki, H.; Toniolo, A.; Notkins, A.L.: Virus-induced diabetes: cytomegalovirus and multiple environmental insults. Diabetologia *24:* 218–219 (1983).
31 Rayfield, E.J.; Seto, Y.; Walsh, S.; McEvoy, R.C.: Virus-induced alterations in insulin release in hamster islets of Langerhans. J. clin. Invest. *68:* 1172–1181 (1981).
32 Prince, G.A.; Jenson, A.B.; Billups, L.C.; Notkins, A.L.: Infection of human pancreatic beta cell cultures with mumps virus. Nature *271:* 158–161 (1978).
33 Yoon, J.W.; Onodera, T.; Jenson, A.B.; Notkins, A.L.: Virus-induced diabetes mellitus. XI. Replication of Coxsackie B3 virus in human pancreatic beta cell cultures. Diabetes *27:* 778–781 (1978).
34 Yoon, J.W.; Selvaggio, S.; Onodera, T.; Wheeler, J.; Jenson, A.B.: Infection of cultured human pancreatic B cells with reovirus type 3. Diabetologia *20:* 462–467 (1981).
35 Jenson, A.B.; Rosenberg, H.S.; Notkins, A.L.: Pancreatic islet cell damage in children with fatal viral infections. Lancet *ii:* 354–358 (1980).
36 Jenson, A.B.; Rosenberg, H.S.: Multiple viruses in diabetes mellitus. Prog. med. Virol., vol. 29, pp. 197–217 (1984).
37 Ujevich, M.M.; Jaffe, R.: Pancreatic islet cell damage. Its occurrence in neonatal Coxsackievirus encephalomyocarditis. Archs Pathol. Lab. Med. *104:* 438–441 (1980).
38 Kaplan, M.H.; Klein, S.W.; McPhee, J.; Harper, R.G.: Group B Coxsackievirus infections in infants younger than three months of age: a serious childhood illness. Rev. infect. Dis. *5:* 1019–1032 (1983).
39 Millard, P.R.: AIDS: histopathological aspects. J. Path. *143:* 223–239 (1984).
40 Patterson, K.; Chandra, R.S.; Jenson, A.B.: Congenital rubella, insulitis, and diabetes mellitus in an infant. Lancet *i:* 1048–1049 (1981).
41 Yoon, J.W.; Austin, M.; Onodera, T.; Notkins, A.L.: Virus-induced diabetes mellitus: isolation of a virus from the pancreas of a child with diabetic ketoacidosis. New Engl. J. Med. *300:* 1173–1179 (1979).
42 Champsaur, H.F.; Bottazzo, G.F.; Bertrams, J.; Assan, R.; Bach, C.: Virologic, immunologic, and genetic factors in insulin-dependent diabetes mellitus. J. Pediat. *100:* 15–20 (1982).
43 Gladisch, R.; Hofmann, W.; Waldherr, R.: Myokarditis and Insulitis nach Coxsackie-Virus Infekt. Z. Kardiol. *65:* 837–849 (1976).
44 Wilson, C.; Connolly, J.H.; Thomson, D.: Coxsackie B2 virus infection and acute-onset diabetes in a child. Br. med. J. *i:* 1007–1008 (1977).
45 Nelson, P.G.; Arthur, L.J.H.; Gurling, K.J.; Gamble, D.R.; Taylor, K.W.: Familial juvenile onset diabetes. Br. med. J. *ii:* 1126–1127 (1977).
46 Kanazawa, Y.: Some genetic and immunological aspects of type I (insulin-dependent) diabetes in Japan; in Andreani, Di Mario, Federlin, Heding, Immunology in diabetes, pp. 159–169 (Kimpton, London 1984).
47 Menser, M.A.; Forrest, J.M.; Bransby, R.D.: Rubella infection and diabetes mellitus. Lancet *i:* 57–60 (1978).
48 Rubinstein, P.; Walker, M.E.; Fedun, B.; Witt, M.E.; Cooper, L.Z.; Ginsberg-Fellner, F.: The HLA system in congenital rubella patients with and without diabetes. Diabetes *31:* 1088–1091 (1982).

49 Ginsberg-Fellner, F.; Witt, M.E.; Yagihashi, S.; Dobersen, M.J.; Taub, F.; Fedun, B.; McEvoy, R.C.; Roman, S.H.; Davies, T.F.; Cooper, L.Z.; Rubinstein, P.; Notkins, A.L.: Congenital rubella syndrome as a model for type 1 (insulin-dependent) diabetes mellitus: increased prevalence of islet cell surface antibodies. Diabetologia *27:* 87–89 (1984).
50 Bottazzo, G.F.; Pujol-Borrel, R.; Hanafusa, T.; Feldmann, M.: Role of aberrant HLA-DR expression and antigen presentation in induction of endocrine autoimmunity. Lancet *ii:* 1115–1119 (1983).
51 Londei, M.; Lamb, J.R.; Bottazzo, G.F.; Feldmann, M.: Epithelial cells expressing aberrant MHC class II determinants can present antigen to cloned human T lymphocytes. Nature *312:* 639–641 (1984).
52 Notkins, A.L.; Onodera, T.; Prabhakar, B.: Virus-induced autoimmunity; in Notkins, Oldstone, Concepts in viral pathogenesis, pp. 210–215 (Springer, New York 1984).
53 Garzelli, C.; Taub, F.E.; Scharff, J.E.; Prabhakar, B.S.; Ginsberg-Fellner, F.; Notkins, A.L.: Epstein-Barr virus-transformed lymphocytes produce monoclonal autoantibodies that react with antigens in multiple organs. J. Virol. *52:* 722–725 (1984).
54 Norden, C.W.; Kuller, L.H.: Identifying infectious etiologies of chronic disease. Rev. infect. Dis. *6:* 200–213 (1984).
55 Christau, B.; Kromann, H.; Anderson, O.O.; Christy, M.; Buschard, K.; Arnung, K.; Kristensen, I.H.; Peitersen, B.; Steinrud, J.; Nerup, J.: Incidence, seasonal and geographical patterns of juvenile-onset insulin-dependent diabetes mellitus in Denmark. Diabetologia *13:* 281–284 (1977).
56 Fleeger, F.M.; Rogers, K.D.; Drash, A.; Rosenbloom, A.L.; Travis, L.B.; Court, J.M.: Age, sex, and season of onset of juvenile diabetes in different geographic areas. Pediatrics *63:* 374–379 (1979).
57 Gamble, D.R.; Kinsley, M.L.; Fitzgerald, M.G.; Bolton, R.; Taylor, K.W.: Viral antibodies in diabetes mellitus. Br. med. J. *iii:* 627–630 (1969).
58 Gamble, D.R.; Taylor, K.W.; Cumming, H.: Coxsackie viruses and diabetes mellitus. Br. med. J. *iv:* 260–262 (1973).
59 Hazra, D.K.; Singh, R.; Wahal, P.K.; Lahiri, V.; Gupta, M.K.; Jain, N.K.; Elhence, B.R.: Coxsackie antibodies in young Asian diabetics. Lancet *i:* 877 (1980).
60 Lozovskaya, L.S.; Desyatskova, R.G.; Smirnoff, V.V.; Sadelkina, L.V.; Shigina, O.M.; Mazurina, N.A.: Antibodies to the rubella virus in the dynamics of juvenile diabetes mellitus. Pediatria *9:* 7–12 (1978).
61 Nelson, P.G.; Pyke, D.A.; Gamble, D.R.: Viruses and the aetiology of diabetes: a study in identical tweens. Br. med. J. *iv:* 249–251 (1975).
62 Pugliese, A.; Cerutti, F.; Toniolo, A.; Corallini, A.; Tovo, P.A.: Diabete giovanile ed infezione rubeolica. Ital. J. Pediat. *11:* 626–627 (1985).
63 Ryder, E.; Ryder, S.: Human Venezuelan equine encephalitis virus infection and diabetes in Zulia State, Venezuela. J. med. Virol. *11:* 327–332 (1983).
64 Yoon, J.W.; Huang, S.W.; McLaren, N.K.; Wheleer, C.J.; Selvaggio, S.S.; Notkins, A.L.: Antibody to encephalomyocarditis virus in juvenile diabetes. New Engl. J. Med. *297:* 1235–1236 (1977).

Prof. Giuseppe Saggese, MD,
Clinica Pediatrica,
Università di Pisa,
Via Roma 35,
I-56100 Pisa (Italy)

Pediatrician *12:* 194–198 (1983–85)

0300–1245/85/0124–0194$2.75/0

Ophthalmologic Complications of Insulin-Dependent Diabetes mellitus in Children and Adolescents

John I. Malone

Diabetes Center, University of South Florida, Tampa, Fla., USA

Key Words. Diabetic · Adolescence · Retinopathy · Cataracts · Aldose reductase inhibitors

Abstract. Diabetes mellitus is a major cause of visual impairment and blindness. Cataracts and retinal vascular abnormalities (retinopathy) are the major defects occurring in the eyes. The frequency of these defects increases with the duration of diabetes. Many believe that the occurrence of eye disease in children with diabetes is rare. Blurry vision, an early manifestation of cataractogenesis, occurs in nearly all children with diabetes. Retinopathy, which is extremely rare prior to puberty, occurs in 70–90% of adolescents with diabetes of more than 10 years' duration. Proliferative retinopathy and blindness due to diabetes also occur in adolescents. Regular, careful ophthalmologic examinations by retinal specialists are indicated for the adolescents at risk. Those at risk are adolescent females with HLA DR3 and DR4 as well as those with limited joint mobility. Early recognition is essential to prevent the blindness that follows untreated proliferative retinopathy.

Diabetes mellitus is a major cause of visual impairment and blindness. This ranges from recurrent blurry vision which is secondary to osmotic changes in the lens to total opacity of the lens which is the diabetic cataract. A greater concern, however, are the vascular abnormalities that develop in the retina without impairment of vision and progress ultimately to irreversible blindness. The later problem, called diabetic retinopathy, is the leading cause of new cases of blindness in the United States today [1]. It is estimated that 75–90% of individuals with type I insulin-dependent diabetes mellitus will develop diabetic retinopathy during their lifetime [2]. Ten to twelve percent of those individuals with retinopathy are at risk for visual loss. In addition, individuals with diabetes are 1.3 times more likely to develop glaucoma and 1.6 times more likely to develop cataracts than nondiabetic individuals [3]. The natural history of diabetes mellitus indicates that the development of all complications including those involving the eye increase with the duration of clinical diabetes. Most physicians are involved in the care of the occasional child with diabetes, it is therefore with limited experience that most have encountered a child with complications other than hypoglycemia and/or diabetic ketoacidosis. For this reason there has been little concern about the evolution of diabetes-associated eye disease during childhood and adolescence. It is important, however, for pediatricians to be aware that the early stages of diabetic eye problems begin during childhood and adolescence. This awareness should direct treatment toward the prevention of the eye complications of diabetes, since current treatment is not effective for reversing these problems once they are established.

Cataracts

The etiology of cataracts in patients with diabetes appears to be directly related to the degree of blood glucose control. Cataracts were noted to be associated with diabetes as early as 1890 [4]. In 1934 a report indicated that 16% of children with insulin-dependent diabetes between the ages of 2 and 33 years had cataracts [4]. The average blood glucose level of those children with cataracts was significantly greater than that of the children who did not have cataracts at the time of the examination. Thus, poorly controlled diabetes mellitus does constitute a cataractogenic factor. Much of our understanding about the association of diabetes to cataract formation has come from studies of animals with experimental diabetes. It has been shown that the lens of rats with experimental diabetes accumulates high levels of sorbitol and fructose [5]. This occurs because of increased activity in the lens of a minor pathway of glucose metabolism the polyol pathway which converts glucose to sorbitol and sorbitol to fructose. *Kinoshita* [6] and associates have shown that excessive accumulation of sorbitol in the lens leads to an increase in intracellular osmolarity, which causes an influx of water with resultant swelling of the lens fibrils. This swelling leads to leakage of glutathione, amino acids and altered membrane permeability, which allows the electrolyte composition of the lens to approach that of the extracellular fluids which finally results in lens opacification. Supporting evidence for this mechanism of cataract formation was provided when compounds which inhibit the first enzyme in the polyol pathway, aldose reductase, prevented cataract formation [7]. Aldose reductase converts the excess glucose of diabetes mellitus to sorbitol which does not cross cell membranes and accumulates intracellularly. This accumulation results in increased tissue water and swelling that causes lens fibril disruption and cataract formation. Thus, lower intracellular levels of glucose, sorbitol, and fructose may be very effective for preventing cataract formation by reducing the excess osmolar burden. Further support for this mechanism comes from the current clinical experience which indicates that cataract formation in young children with diabetes is currently at a level much below the 16% reported earlier when blood glucose levels were not controlled as well as they are today.

The degree of blood glucose control that is achievable in most children today has apparently reduced the frequency of cataract formation but has not eliminated the common problem of changes in refractive index (blurry vision) caused by osmotic changes in the lens in response to unstable blood glucose levels. These fluctuations in the blood glucose value lead to visual difficulties for school children who are unable to see the blackboard in school and are also unable to get a satisfactory refraction of their eyes when they visit their ophthalmologist. Blurry vision is usually troublesome for the child and should be a motivator for improved metabolic control on the part of the patient.

Clinical experience indicates that the appearance of cataracts is a late manifestation of diabetes. The early ocular manifestations of cataractogenesis consist of ametropia which can be either hyperametropia or myopia [8]. It has been demonstrated that the ametropic changes in diabetic subjects is a consequence primarily of alterations in the lens refractive index. Studies using experimentally induced diabetes in rabbits have shown that the ametropic changes are initiated by the accumulation of sorbitol in the lens. The changes in the refractive index produced by diabetes can be returned to normal with the use of an aldose reductase inhibitor [9]. Animal experiments indicate that near normalization of the blood glucose can prevent changes in refractive index which cause blurry vision and will also prevent the cataracts associated with the long-term hyperglycemia of diabetes mellitus. Since there are practical problems associated with achieving this ideal control of blood glucose, a second possibility of current interest is the use of aldose reductase inhibitors. An inhibitor that is currently being tested in the US and Europe is sorbinil. Animal studies indicate that red cell sorbitol values reflect lens sorbitol levels [10]. Many clinical trials have shown that sorbinil is effective for returning red cell sorbitol levels in human diabetics to normal [10]. Thus, one would assume that this aldose reductase inhibitor would prevent cataract formation in humans as it does in animals with experimental diabetes.

Retinopathy

Diabetic retinopathy is a microvascular complication of diabetes mellitus. The retinal vascular lesions of diabetes seem to progress with duration of the disease from a low of 2.5 cases per 100 after 10 years of diabetes to 90 cases per 100 following 30 years of diabetes [2]. Histologically, the vascular changes include the loss of capillary pericytes, the accumulation of endothelial cells, and thickening of the vascular basement membrane with occlusion of the capillary lumen, development of compensatory shunt vessels and dilation of the capillaries. The dilated capillaries are thin-walled and leak erythrocytes which are seen as small hemorrhages. Red blood cells in the dilated capillaries and the small hemorrhages are perceived as microaneurysms which are the earliest vascular abnormalities recognized by direct light visualization. These changes may progress in certain individuals to new vessel formation, larger hemorrhages, fluid exudation, and retinal detachment, which are well-recognized stages of diabetic retinopathy. When these vascular changes are well developed they can be observed with an ophthalmoscope. Retinopathy was first observed in the late 1800s soon after the ophthalmoscope was developed [11]. This condition, however, was only rarely seen prior to the 1940s and most observations of diabetic retinopathy have been made since that time. Between 1958 and 1962, *Sorsby* [12] found that approximately 7% of the new cases of blindness registered in the United Kingdom were due to diabetic retinopathy. By 1968 that figure had increased to 13.1% of all new cases of blindness [13]. A report from the Joslin Clinic in 1976 indicated that 12% of the individuals followed for 40 years with insulin-dependent diabetes were legally blind from diabetic retinopathy [14]. The highest reported figure to date is 23% of all registrations for blindness in Denmark were due to diabetic retinopathy during the period from 1958 through 1961 [15]. It is important to understand that the risk for progressing from good vision to blindness depends upon the type of retinopathy present. If an individual has background retinopathy which is scattered microaneurysms without new vessel formation, the risk for blindness during the next 5 years approaches zero [16]. If hemorrhage and exudates are present, the risk for blindness increases to 4% during the succeeding 5 years. The visual prognosis is much worse if new vessels are present. If one has good vision and four or fewer areas of neovascularization with no fibrous proliferation or vitreous hemorrhage, then 4% of those individuals will become blind within 1 year. If the new vessel formation is more extensive and fibrous proliferation and vitreous hemorrhage are absent, the prognosis is worse with 14% becoming blind in 1 year. If both fibrous proliferation and vitreous hemorrhage exist, the chance of blindness increases to 37% in 1 year. It is important to distinguish between proliferative retinopathy (neovascularization) and background retinopathy (scattered areas of microaneurysms) when discussing diabetic retinopathy. Those reports which indicate that 75–90% of young people with type I diabetes have retinopathy should not be interpreted as indicating that all of these individuals have a high risk of progression to blindness. Only those who develop neovascular changes in the retina have a high risk of blindness and, based on the information provided above, this seems to account for 10–12% of those individuals who have diabetes. The diabetic retinopathy study conducted by the National Institutes of Health demonstrated that retinal photocoagulation can delay or prevent severe visual loss in more than 50% of eyes with proliferative retinopathy [17]. Thus, appropriate diagnosis is important to allow monitoring of the evolution of retinopathy so that photocoagulation can be applied at the appropriate time if necessary. Using the direct ophthalmoscope, the vascular changes of diabetes have not been noted in the eyes of children less than 10 years of age. Surveys of insulin-dependent diabetics less than 20 years of age have revealed only a 7% incidence of diabetic retinopathy [18]. A more sensitive method for detecting the earliest vascular changes is the use of sodium fluorescein prior to the photographic recording of the retinal vessels (fig. 1). This technique allows careful evaluation of the anatomy of the retinal capillaries and therefore is a more sensitive indicator of vascular abnormalities [19]. Using this technique, various investigators have reported an incidence of diabetic retinopathy in children with diabetes of less than 5 years' duration ranging from 1 to 18% (table I) [20]. The same investigators have noted vascular abnormalities ranging in frequency from 20 to 56% in children with diabetes of 6–10 years' duration. After 10 years of diabetes most investigators agree upon a high frequency of retinopathy ranging from 70 to 90%. During a 4- to 6-year longitudinal study [20] of 74 children with insulin-dependent diabetes, we observed 11 of those individuals progress to proliferative diabetic retinopathy requiring laser photocoagulation before the age of 21 years. Of this group, 2 progressed to legal blindness – one at the age of 18 and the other at the age of 20 years. During this study we identified significant retinopathy using fluorescein angiography in young people who ranged in age from 9 to 21 years with diabetes duration ranging from 5 to 14 years. One child developed obvious vascular abnormalities prior to the onset of puberty at 9 years of age. The youngest individual developing proliferative retinopathy requiring laser photocoagulation was 16 years of age. Although the frequency of retinopathy in children of this age is small, the incidence in this study indicates that careful evaluation of the eyes of children with diabetes is an important aspect of the quality management of diabetes in children.

Table I. Retinopathy studies of youth with retinopathy defined by fluorescein angiography

Duration years	*Malone* et al. [21]	*Palmberg* et al. [22]	*Frank* et al. [23]	*Dorchy* et al. [24]
<5	19/104 (18)	10/107 (9)	1/77 (1)	5/39 (13)
6–10	9/40 (22)	39/73 (53)	16/71 (23)	17/31 (56)
11–16	7/10 (70)	37/45 (82)	12/18 (67)	15/17 (88)

Values shown are the number of positive studies/total number of studies. Figures in parentheses are percentages.

There are certain factors that help identify those individuals at greatest risk for developing retinopathy with diabetes of short duration. Our 4- to 6-year follow-up of children indicated that those individuals with the greatest risk of developing proliferative retinopathy are teenage females with the HLA type DR3 and 4 [20]. The risk of developing observable retinopathy prior to the onset of puberty is highly unlikely. After puberty the risk is significant and it increases with the duration of diabetes. If one has diabetes for 10 years and is postpubertal, the risk of having retinopathy is greater than 80%. *Rosenbloom* et al. [25] have also noted that children with diabetes who have limited joint mobility are at increased risk for having diabetic retinopathy. They report that children with diabetes for more than 16 years who have limited joint mobility have an 83% risk for retinopathy while those without limited joint mobility have only a 25% risk. Thus, physicians caring for adolescents with diabetes and limited joint mobility must be certain that their patients have regular ophthalmologic evaluations.

Regular ophthalmologic evaluations are an essential part of the medical care plan. It is important that the physician evaluating the eyes be trained and aware of the retinal problems that are of concern. One report indicates [26] that 61% of patients with diabetic retinopathy were missed by a group of senior medical residents, board certified internists and diabetologists asked to specifically examine patients for diabetic retinopathy using direct ophthalmoscopy. This report also indicated that proliferative retinopathy was missed by 52% of the internists, 50% of the senior medical residents, 33% of the diabetologists and 9% of the general ophthalmologists. None of the retina specialists missed proliferative retinopathy. Since accurate early diagnosis is important for avoiding the blindness caused by unrecognized proliferative retinopathy, careful selection of the ophthalmology consultant is essential.

The current understanding and treatment of diabetic retinopathy remains very rudimentary. Two recent animal studies suggest, however, that the polyol pathway may also be involved in the pathogenesis of these retinal vascular abnormalities. *Engerman and Kern* [27] have shown that normal dogs with dietarily induced elevation of the hexose galactose develop capillary aneurysms and other retinal lesions like those characteristic of diabetes mellitus. These dogs with normal blood glucose, lipids, branch chain amino acids and serum insulin levels developed retinopathy after being fed galactose for 32 months. This suggests that elevated concentrations of hexoses (i.e. galactose and glucose) can be etiologic in the evolution of

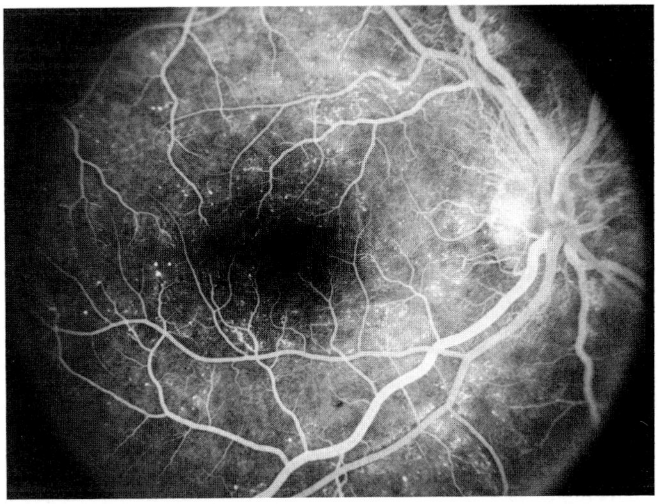

Fig. 1. Fluorescein angiogram photograph of the retina of the right eye in a 16-year-old female with insulin-dependent diabetes mellitus of 4 years duration. The macula is in the center and the optic disc to the right. The angiogram shows a black dot just above the major venule crossing the lower ⅓ of the retina. This area is black because fluorescein was excluded.

diabetic-like retinopathy. This observation coupled with the report of *Robison* et al. [28] that galactose-induced retinopathy in the rat can be prevented by the aldose reductase inhibitor, sorbinil, suggests that the polyol pathway may also play a role in the pathogenesis of diabetic associated microvasculopathy. To date, these very encouraging laboratory investigations have not been confirmed in human diabetes, but clinical trials are currently being conducted by the National Eye Institute [29] to determine if aldose reductase inhibitors might play a role in preventing diabetic retinopathy.

In conclusion, eye disease associated with diabetes does cause significant morbidity in the lives of adolescents and young adults. Physicians caring for these young people must be aware of the potential hazard and encourage a high degree of metabolic control in these individuals, particularly those females who are HLA DR3 and DR4. The current therapy for these problems as they evolve is very limited and destructive in the form of laser photocoagulation. It is hoped that the suggested benefit of aldose reductase inhibitors in laboratory animals will have practical application in humans and this medical approach would be highly desirable since it would prevent the development of the pathologic condition. The ultimate treatment will be the total reversal of the abnormal metabolism of diabetes mellitus – a cure!

References

1 Diabetes: 1985 annual report national diabetes advisory board. NIH Publ. No. 85–1587, p. 6 (US Department of Health and Human Services, Bethesda, Md. 1985).

2 White, P.: The child with diabetes. Med. Clins N. Am. *49:* 1069–1079 (1965).

3 US Department of Health and Human Services: Screening for diabetic eye disease – Mississippi. Morbid. Mortal. Wkly Rep. *32:* 157–158 (1983).

4 Varma, S.D.; Richards, R.D.: Etiology of cataracts in diabetics; in Pavan, Ocular manifestations of diabetes. Int. Ophthal. Clins *24:* 93–110 (1984).

5 Van Heyningen, R.: Formation of polyols by the lens of the rat with sugar cataracts. Nature *184:* 194–195 (1959).

6 Kinoshita, J.H.: Cataracts in galactosemia. Investve Ophthal. vis. Sci. *4:* 786–789 (1965).

7 Varma, S.D.; Kinoshita, J.H.: Inhibition of lens aldose reductase by flavenoids – their possible role in the prevention of diabetic cataract. Biochem. Pharmac. *25:* 2505–2513 (1976).

8 Eversman, J.: Comprehensive approach to diabetes mellitus. Aud. Dig. intern. Med. *18:* 23 (1971).

9 Varma, S.D.; Schocket, S.S.; Richards, R.D.: Implications of aldose reductase in cataracts in human diabetes. Investve Ophthal. vis. Sci. *18:* 237–241 (1979).

10 Malone, J.I.; Leavengood, H.; Peterson, M.J.; Obrien, M.M.; Page, M.G.; Aldinger, C.E.: Red blood cell sorbitol as an indicator of polyol pathway activity. Diabetes *33:* 45–49 (1984).

11 Jaeger, E.: Ophthalmoskopischer Hand-Atlas, p. 99 (K.K. Hof- und Staatsdruckerei, Wien 1869).

12 Sorsby, A.: The incidence and causes of blindness in England and Wales 1948–1962. Reports on public health and medical subjects, No. 114 (Her Majesty's Stationery Office, London 1966).

13 Sorsby, A.: The incidence and causes of blindness in England and Wales 1963–1968. Reports on public health and medical subjects, No. 28, pp. 33, 51 (Her Majesty's Stationery Office, London 1972).

14 Paz-Guevara, A.T.; Tah-Hsiung Hsu; White, P.: Juvenile diabetes mellitus after forty years. Diabetes *24:* 559–565 (1975).

15 Vedel-Jensen, N.: Dan. med. Bull. *9:* 185 (1962).

16 Kohner, E.M.; McLeod, D.; Marshall, J.: Diabetic eye disease; in Keen, Jarrett, Complications of diabetes sec, p. 19 (Arnold, London 1982).

17 The Diabetic Retinopathy Study Research Group: Photocoagulation treatment of proliferative diabetic retinopathy. Clinical application of diabetic retinopathy study (DRS) findings. DRS report No. 8. Ophthalmology *88:* 583–600 (1981).

18 Larsen, H.W.: The clinical characteristics of diabetic retinopathy. Proc. Int. Symp. Fluorescein Angiography, pp. 346–355 (Karger, Basel 1971).

19 Davis, M.; de Venecia, G.: Histology and fluorescein angiography of microaneurysms in diabetes mellitus. Proc. Int. Symp. Fluorescein Angiography (Karger, Basel 1971).

20 Malone, J.I.; Grizzard, W.S.; Espinoza, L.R.; Achenbach, K.E.; Van Cader, T.C.: Risk factors for diabetic retinopathy in youth. Pediatrics *73:* 756–761 (1984).

21 Malone, J.I.; Van Cader, T.C.; Edwards, W.C.: Diabetes vascular changes in children. Diabetes *26:* 673–679 (1977).

22 Palmberg, P.; Smith, M.; Waltman, S.; Krupin, T.; Singer, P.; Burgess, D.; Wendtlant, T.; Achtenberg, J.; Cryer, P.; Santiago, J.; White, N.; Kilo, C.; Daughaday, W.: The natural history of retinopathy in insulin dependent juvenile onset diabetes. Ophthalmology *88:* 613–618 (1981).

23 Frank, R.N.; Hoffman, W.H.; Podgor, M.J.; Joondeph, H.C.; Lewis, R.A.; Margherio, R.R.; Nachazel, D.P.; Weiss, H.; Christopherson, K.W.; Cronin, M.A.: Retinopathy in juvenile onset type I diabetes of short duration. Diabetes *31:* 874–882 (1982).

24 Dorchy, H.; Toussaint, D.; Devroede, M.; Ernould, C.; Loeb, H.: Diagnostic de la rétinopathie diabétique infantile par angiographie fluorescéinique. Nouv. Presse méd. *6:* 345–347 (1977).

25 Rosenbloom, A.L.; Silverstein, J.H.; Lezotte, D.C.; Richardson, K.; McCallum, M.: Limited joint mobility in childhood diabetes mellitus indicates increased risk for microvascular disease. New Engl. J. Med. *305:* 191–194 (1981).

26 Sussman, E.J.; Tsiaras, W.G.; Soper, K.A.: Diagnosis of diabetic eye disease. J. Am. med. Ass. *247:* 3231–3234 (1982).

27 Engerman, R.L.; Kern, T.S.: Experimental galactosemia produces diabetic-like retinopathy. Diabetes *33:* 97–100 (1984).

28 Robison, W.G.; Kador, P.F.; Kinoshita, J.H.: Retinal capillaries: basement membrane thickening by galactosemia prevented with aldose reductase inhibitor. Science *221:* 1177–1179 (1983).

29 Marwick, C.: NIH testing sorbinil to prevent retinopathy. J. Am. med. Ass. *252:* 1263 (1984).

Received: November 4, 1985

John I. Malone, MD,
Professor of Pediatrics,
Co-Director, University of South Florida,
Diabetes Center,
Tampa, FL 33612 (USA)

Pediatrician *12:* 199–207 (1983–85)

0300–1245/85/0124–0199$2.75/0

Etiology, Diagnosis, and Prevention of Renal Involvement in Insulin-Dependent Diabetes mellitus

Giuseppe Chiumello, Luciano Beccaria, Franco Meschi, Laila Mistura, Paolo Brambilla, Emilio Bognetti

Pediatric Department, Endocrine Unit, University of Milano, Italy

Key Words. Diabetic nephropathy · Diabetic complications · Type 1 diabetes mellitus

Abstract. Overt diabetic nephropathy is a well-established clinical picture characterized by macroproteinuria and irreversible decline of glomerular function. The first phase of renal involvement has been widely investigated in the last decade in the hope to individuate early lesions. Five stages of glomerular damage have been identified by morphological abnormalities and clinical tests. Although renal hypertrophy, hyperfiltration, and microalbuminuria are present in all diabetics at onset, subsequent evolution shows different patterns: some patients may present no further progression, while others show a rapid and irreversible decline of kidney function. This suggests that other factors, i.e., risk factors, may play important roles in the renal involvement in diabetics. The predictive role of microalbuminuria and of hyperfiltration was investigated, and, so far, only an albumin excretion rate above 30 μg/min has been proved to be associated with a decline of renal function. Actually no practical hints can be given to prevent the disease apart from persistent strict glycometabolic control during the course of diabetes. Antihypertensive treatment can slow glomerular damage when overt diabetic nephropathy and hypertension are present. Aggressive treatment in the early phases of renal involvement might change the natural history of the disease.

Introduction

Diabetic nephropathy is an important complication of diabetes mellitus characterized by abnormal albumin excretion rate (AER), persistently above 0.5 g/day, hypertension, and morphological structural glomerular abnormalities. These findings are associated with a progressive and irreversible decline of kidney function with progressive reduction of glomerular filtration rate (GFR) up to end-stage renal failure. Current therapeutic tools only reduce the rate of decline of GFR, but do not arrest the fatal evolution [1, 2].

About 40% of insulin-dependent diabetic patients and about half of diabetic children will develop diabetic nephropathy with a peak incidence after 16 years of disease [3, 4]; the risk of developing diabetic nephropathy seems lower for patients with a duration of the disease over 35 years [3].

Several studies have shown that structural and morphological abnormalities – mesangial matrix and glomerular basement membrane (GBM) thickening – are found in every long-term type 1 diabetic patient [5], though only a few develop overt diabetic nephropathy. So minimal glomerular alterations seem to be a hallmark of diabetes mellitus, while the evolution toward overt nephropathy seems to be a complication arising only in some patients through unexplained mechanisms.

Five stages of clinical and morphological alterations of kidney function and structure during the course of diabetes mellitus can be identified now (table I).

Stage one, called 'early hypertrophy hyperfunction', is only observed at the onset of diabetes mellitus. Newly diagnosed diabetic patients without insulin therapy show increased GFR and AER both at rest and after physical exercise, but normal renal plasma flow (RPF) and β_2-microglobulin excretion [6, 7]. These findings are indica-

Table I. Staging of diabetic nephropathy

Stage	Chronology	GFR	RPF	AER		Selectivity index[1]	Blood pressure	Morphological changes	Therapeutical approach
				basal	after exercise				
1	at diagnosis (usually improves with good control)	increased by 20–40%	normal or slightly increased	increased (micro-albuminuria)	increased	low	normal	kidney enlargement, nephron hypertrophy, normal thickness of GBM	strict glycometabolic control
2	long-term diabetics (after 2 years of disease)	increased (20%)	normal or slightly increased	normal	increased in some patients	high (0.6)	normal	increased thickness of GBM, initial mesangial expansion	progress to overt nephropathy in 40–50% of patients, the efficacy of strict control is unknown
3	long-term diabetics	increased (20–30%)	slow decline	micro-albuminuria (30–150 or 15–300 μg/min)	increased	low (0.2)	increased or sometimes in normal range	unknown	to be investigated
4	long-term diabetics (maximum incidence after 16 years of disease)	decline (approximately 1 ml/min/month)	decline (approximately 5 ml/min/month)	macro-proteinuria (Albustix positive)	increased	low (0.2)	increased	glomerulosclerosis of Kimmelstein-Wilson	strict blood pressure control and good metabolic control slow the progression
5	approximately 5 years after appearance of clinical proteinuria	< 10 ml/min	low	macro-proteinuria	–	high (0.6)	elevated	diffuse glomerular sclerosis	dialysis

For explanation see Introduction.
[1] Clearance IgG/clearance albumin.

tive of abnormalities of glomerular function with normal tubular function. Kidney enlargement has been well documented by ultrasound or X-ray techniques [8, 9]. The improved metabolic control with the start of insulin therapy can restore normal AER both at rest and after exercise within 2 weeks [7, 10] and within 3 months both GFR and kidney volume [11]. Microscopic studies during the early phase of diabetes mellitus have shown minimal glomerular abnormalities such as increased mean capillary volume and increased glomerular volume, but a normal thickness of the GBM [12, 13].

Stage two is seen in long-term diabetic patients. For many years after starting insulin therapy, during standard controls, characteristically all standard clinical parameters related to renal function are normal. However, some diabetic patients present increased GFR and kidney enlargement [14, 15], but normal AER and β_2-microglobulin excretion at rest [16, 17], with a minimal increment in AER (microalbuminuria) after physical exercise [16, 17]. Morphological glomerular abnormalities at this stage are increased thickness of the GBM and increased mesangial matrix with deposition of mesangial membrane-like material [18]. A large number of patients will have only these abnormalities for a long time with no progression, but some of them (about 40%) will move on to the next stages for reasons currently unknown.

Stage three is a well-defined new entity known as 'incipient diabetic nephropathy', characterized by a slight increase of AER (microalbuminuria) both at rest and after exercise, with β_2-microglobulin excretion still in the normal range. The GFR may be elevated, and the blood pressure may be slightly higher, though in the normal range [7]. Few histological studies have been done in this stage, and an increased thickness of the epithelial foot processes is the only reported difference from the previous stage [19].

Stage four is characterized by overt clinical nephropathy with persistent macroproteinuria (over 0.5 g/day; Albustix positive). The GFR may be normal or even supranormal, but at the beginning of this stage it may progressively decline at a rate of about 1 ml/min/month [20] up to end-stage renal failure in a few years (5–7 years) [3]. β_2-Microglobulin excretion progressively rises [20], probably owing to inhibition of the reabsorption process by competition from other proteins filtered, due to glomerular lesions. In these patients thickening of the GBM, increased mesangial volume, and deposition of mesangial membrane-like material and plasma proteins are more evident. Focal mesangial thickening of PAS-positive material (nodular glomerulosclerosis of Kimmelstein-Wilson), afferent-efferent arteriolar hyalinosis, and linear extracellular glomerular membrane deposition of plasma proteins (IgG, IgM, albumin) are also present [18, 21].

Stage five is the terminal stage and is at present the inevitable destiny of overt diabetic nephropathy characterized by very low GFR (10–15 ml/min). Patients need dialytic therapy and kidney transplantation.

Etiopathogenesis

Only part of the insulin-dependent diabetic population will develop diabetic nephropathy, while the majority seems to be protected from it, developing only minimal changes. The reasons for this are still unknwon, and over the past 20 years, several investigators have worked to clarify them. The roles of glomerular hyperfiltration and microalbuminuria have been analyzed as important factors in the pathogenesis of diabetic nephropathy.

In newly diagnosed diabetic patients the GFR is abnormally elevated [6], and in 25–40% of long-term diabetic patients the GFR is about 40% higher than normal [15]. Multiple factors are involved in this elevation of the GFR in diabetic patients.

The GFR is physiologically the result of the ultrafiltration pressure and the ultrafiltration coefficient. The ultrafiltration coefficient depends on intrinsic characteristics and on the size of the filtration surface. It is well known that newly diagnosed diabetic patients have an increased filtration surface (hypertrophy) [8, 9, 22] responsible, at least in part, for the GFR abnormalities of early diabetes. However, some long-term diabetic patients have an elevated GFR despite normal kidney volume [15]. Furthermore, insulin therapy in newly diagnosed insulin-dependent diabetic patients can correct the GFR within about 1 week [9], but correction of the kidney volume takes 3 months [8]. These factors indicate that the kidney enlargement may play an important role in the pathogenesis of hyperfiltration, but factors other than kidney volume are involved in the glomerular hyperfiltration.

Ultrafiltration pressure is positively related to intraglomerular pressure and negatively to oncotic pressure. While the latter is unchanged [23], the former has been reported to be abnormal in diabetes. In fact, both in newly diagnosed and in long-term diabetics, an increase of ultrafiltration pressure has been documented [24–26].

Other factors may affect GFR in diabetic patients. The high blood glucose level per se has been considered. In normal subjects intravenous glucose infusion can slightly raise the GFR [27]. Furthermore, a correlation between blood glucose level and GFR has been documented in patients with mild hyperglycemia [15]. Intravenous insulin infusion can reduce the GFR in diabetics, but this effect is suppressed by simultaneous glucose infusion [28].

High growth hormone and glucagon levels, usually found in diabetic patients, have been reported to play a role in the pathogenesis of hyperfiltration [29, 30]. High levels of plasma renin activity are reported in diabetes with elevated GFR after physical exercise [31]; it has been suggested that the abnormal response of the renin-angiotensin system to a high level of prostaglandins, or an insensitivity of renal arterioles to angiotensin, may be involved in raising the GFR.

In the last few years the role of glomerular hyperfiltration as a factor in the pathogenesis of glomerular damages has been widely investigated. Experimental studies have shown a direct relationship between glomerular hyperfiltration and the rate of glomerulosclerosis. In fact, in diabetic and normal animals with extensive nephrectomy [32, 33] as well as in patients with unilateral renal agenesis [34], the sclerosis of residual nephrons seems to be accelerated. How glomerular hyperfiltration can worsen glomerulosclerosis is still debated. It has been suggested that the increased intraglomerular pressure could stimulate mesangial proliferation and subsequently aggravate glomerulosclerosis both through direct mechanical stress and increased filtration of plasma proteins into the GBM and the mesangium [35]. The progressive closure of nephrons leads to an increased pressure load in the residual nephrons with accelerated destruction of the glomeruli (table II).

Different levels of microalbuminuria up to macroalbuminuria are often present during the course of diabetes mellitus [36]. New sensitive radioimmunological methods for measuring low urinary albumin concentrations have made it possible to study this parameter in the various stages of diabetes mellitus, particularly the early stages. AER has proved to be one of the most important parameters for studying progressive diabetic renal damage, particularly the 'status' of the glomerular filter.

The GBM is the barrier between blood and urine and can be visualized like a filter with 55-ångström diameter pores uniformly coated by negative charges in a constant interaction with plasma proteins [37]. The size and the electric charges of the plasma molecules, the glomerular

Table II. Role of hyperfiltration in the pathogenesis of diabetic nephropathy

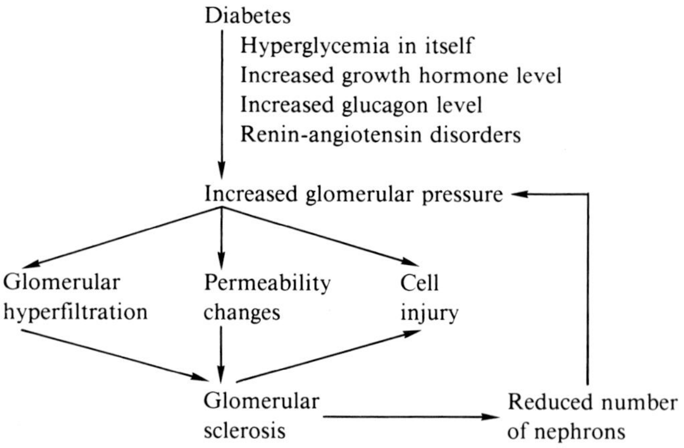

driving forces, and the structure of the GBM are the variables involved in the filtration of plasma proteins by the glomerulus [37].

Plasma albumin is a polyanionic protein with 69,000 daltons and a 36-ångström Stockes radius that crosses the glomerular barrier in a minimal amount due to electric interaction with the glomerular barrier. The minimal amount filtered is then reabsorbed by the renal tubules (97%), and only a very small part escapes into the urine [38]. Other plasma proteins like IgG, an essentially neutral molecule of 160,000 daltons and a 55-ångström Stockes radius, cannot cross the glomerular barrier because it is too big and only a minimal amount escapes into the urine [38]; β_2-microglobulin, a small protein, can cross the glomerular filter freely, but is completely reabsorbed by the tubules [39]. Abnormalitie in the glomerular electric charges will result in increased AER; meanwhile, an abnormal diameter or number of the pores will increase IgG excretion more than the AER. An increase in AER, IgG, and β_2-microglobulin excretion rate will indicate tubular proteinuria.

An increased albumin and IgG excretion rate with a normal β_2-microglobulin excretion is normally found in microproteinuric diabetic patients [39]. The selectivity index (clearance IgG/clearance albumin) is unchanged with AER of 12–30 μg/min because of the parallel increase of both albumin and IgG excretion [40], indicating that pore size and glomerular electric charges are normal. It has been suggested that microproteinuria may be due to increased intraglomerular pressure [41] or to an increased number of pores (renal hypertrophy) [22]. Both hypotheses have been demonstrated, but the rapid reversibility of microalbuminuria after metabolic improvement [42] indicates that the former mechanism is more important, but is not the only one involved.

A very low selectivity index is found with AER of 60–90 μg/min, as a result of increased AER with normal IgG excretion [40]. In these patients glomerular electric charges are much reduced [43], enhancing only the filtration of polyanionic molecules like albumin, while the urinary excretion of neutral molecules (like IgG) is unchanged.

A progressive increase of IgG is observed in macroproteinuric diabetic patients with overt clinical nephropathy [40] due to structural abnormalities of both glomerular pores and glomerular electric charges. The selectivity index is now still high because of the parallel increase of both albumin and IgG excretion rate. Elevated levels of β_2-microglobulin are present when the GFR falls below 40 ml/min/1.73 m^2 [36], due to saturation of tubular reabsorptive capacity in functioning nephrons with protein load.

Morphological Changes

Diabetic nephropathy is characterized by glomerular abnormalities such as GBM, tubular basement membrane and mesangial thickening, afferent and efferent arteriolar hyalinosis, and linear extracellular plasma protein deposition in GMB, tubular basement membrane, Bowman's membrane, and mesangial matrix [5, 21]. The nodular lesion of Kimmelstein-Wilson, considered itself a diagnostic finding, is present in about 50% of diabetic kidneys and represents advanced focal mesangial thickening of PAS-positive material [5, 21]. In the late phase of diabetic nephropathy a large, diffuse increase of the glomerular components (mesangium and GBM) leads to complete closure of the glomerular tuft [18].

Some abnormalities are already present in the newly diagnosed diabetic patient. Enlargement of the glomerular tuft may be observed due to enlargement of the individual capillary lumen and individual glomerular cells [12]. Quantitative electron microscopic studies have shown that both the amount of mesangial basement membrane-like material and the thickness of peripheral basement membrane are normal [13], but the absolute area of the peripheral basement membrane is increased, like the interface between the tuft and the urinary space [22]. It has been concluded that the rate of GBM synthe-

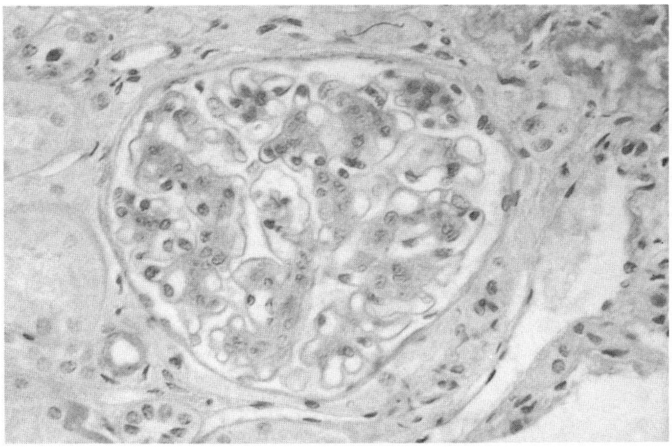

1

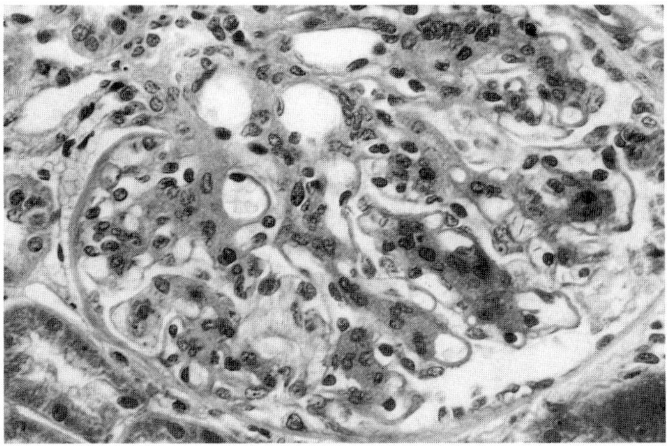

2

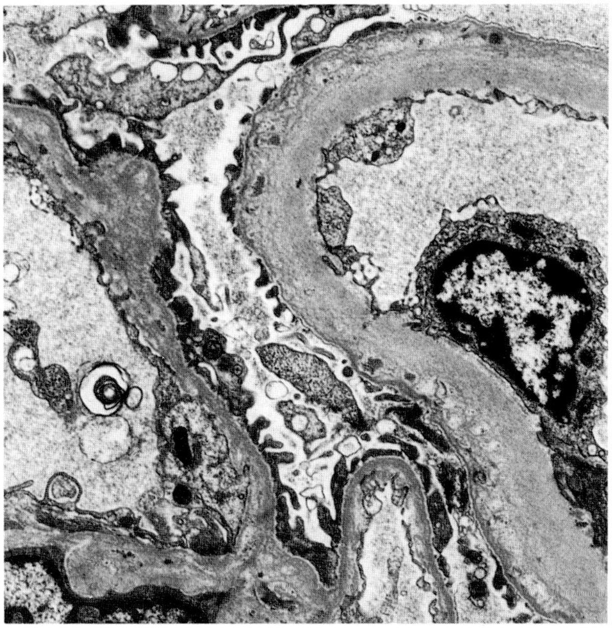

3

Fig. 1. Diffuse diabetic glomerulosclerosis: increased mesangial matrix.

Fig. 2. Diffuse diabetic glomerulosclerosis: increased mesangial matrix and capillary wall thickening.

Fig. 3. Electron microscopic picture of diabetic glomerulosclerosis: glomerular basement membrane thickening.

sis is already high in newly diagnosed diabetic patients because of increased activity of the renal cortex enzyme involved [44].

After some years of diabetes an increase in GBM thickness, associated with increased mesangial volume and capillary volume, has been described [18].

In long-term diabetic patients with diabetic nephropathy the glomerular morphological-structural abnormalities are more advanced. The GBM thickness is doubled compared to the early stages of diabetes, the mesangial region occupies nearly 60% of the total tuft compared to 30% in the early stages, with marked accumulation of basement membrane-like material and renal extracellular basement membrane plasma protein deposition [18, 21].

Figures 1–3 show optic and electron microscopic pictures of glomerular lesions present in a type 1 diabetic adolescent with overt diabetic nephropathy followed in our department.

Diagnosis

Overt diabetic nephropathy is easily diagnosed by clinical tests, but at this stage the possibilities of arresting the natural evolution of the disease towards renal failure are nil. Thus, parameters useful early in the course of diabetes to predict the risk of developing diabetic nephropathy have been studied.

Daily AER was one of the first parameters considered. Basal microalbuminuria has been identified in some type 1 diabetic patients [45, 46], and an increased risk of diabetic nephropathy has been associated with critical levels of microalbuminuria [48]. Longitudinal studies have shown that patients with basal AER of 15–300 μg/min [47] or 30–140 μg/min [48] will develop diabetic nephropathy more frequently than patients with lower values. However, repeated samples and sensitive radioimmunoassay methods are necessary to identify these low urinary albumin concentrations. Short-term AER variability has been clearly shown in normals and diabetics [49], and several factors such as fever, infections, heavy exercise, exposure to cold, and changes in posture can increase AER [50]. So at least three measurements must be made in each patient to identify diabetics with real high-risk microalbuminuria. Some authors have used overnight urine collections to evaluate AER because this method seems free of random variations such as that due to heavy exercise [51]. Daily AER is reported by some authors to be positively correlated to duration of diabetes, puberal stage, and metabolic control, but no general agreement exists about these points [45, 51, 52]. The presence of microalbuminuria in short-term diabetics, even in fair metabolic control, suggests that basal AER measurements should be included in standard routine tests for diabetic children after 5 years of disease. Figure 4 shows daily AER in a group of diabetics followed in our department.

Microalbuminuria after low-grade exercise has been identified in some long-term diabetic children and adolescents with normal AER at rest [16, 17]; so to evaluate latent glomerular abnormalities, AER can be measured after exercise. Figure 5 shows postexercise AER in diabetic children and adolescents studied in our department.

The relationship between postexercise microalbuminuria and clinical features of the patients are still being debated, particularly the relationship with metabolic control [17, 53]. Moreover, the future course of renal involvement in diabetic children with postexercise microalbuminuria is still unpredictable, so basal AER is the only parameter that can actually forecast the evolution of renal damage.

Hyperfiltration in diabetes is well documented in adults [14] and in children with type 1 diabetes [24]. The possible role of this factor in the pathogenesis of diabetic nephropathy has been clearly illustrated by the experimental demonstrations of Brenner et al. [35]. The predictive value of this parameter has still to be definitively confirmed, but it has been recently shown that diabetic patients with a higher GFR showed a faster decline in kidney function than patients with lower GFR. Unfortunately, the hyperfiltering patients also presented microproteinuria [47]. A critical level of GFR has not been identified, but the more marked is renal hyperfiltration, the higher is the risk of developing persistent renal damage. For this reason it is very important to assess this parameter in every diabetic child. Multiple assessments of GFR in cases with diabetic nephropathy can predict

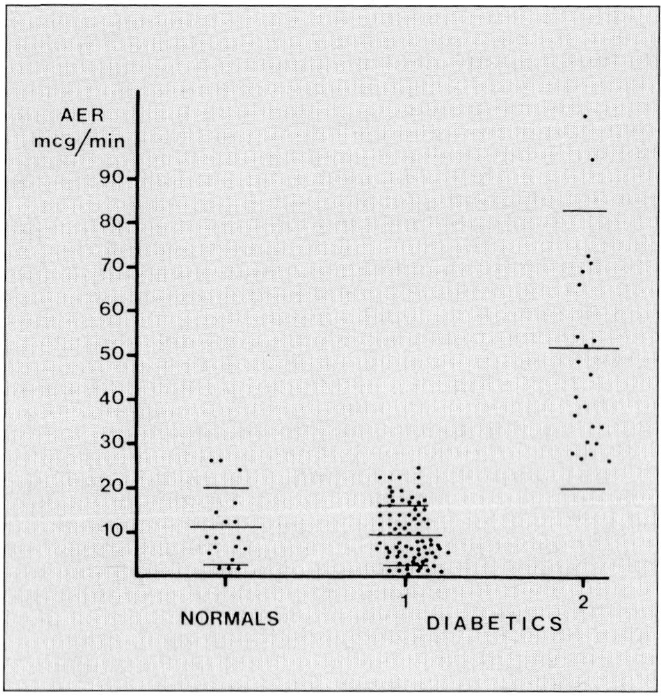

Fig. 4. Basal AER in 18 normal children and in 120 type 1 diabetic children divided into two groups. Group 1 consisted of 98 diabetic children with basal AER in the normal range, and group 2 comprised 22 diabetic children with basal AER above the upper limit of normals. Age, duration of disease, and metabolic control evaluated by HbA1 were not different in the two groups.

the slope of decline in kidney function up to end-stage renal failure [20].

Inulin and *p*-aminohippuric acid clearance are the reference methods for evaluating GFR and RPF, but they are very difficult to perform in children, and simple methods using radioisotopes are now available [54]. Creatinine clearance is often used in clinical studies, but wide variability is seen in the results because of technical errors [55]. So in children, a single injection of radioisotopes or constant inulin infusion offer better results [54, 56].

The kidney volume is often increased in hyperfiltering diabetics [14], and it must be carefully checked, because it is one of the factors involved in the pathogenesis of renal hyperfiltration. Echographic methods are available and give good results [57].

The mean blood pressure is reported to be slightly raised in microalbuminuric patients, but still in the normal range [58]. However, accurate monitoring of the blood pressure can identify early abnormal raises, especially in microproteinuric patients with high-risk AER values.

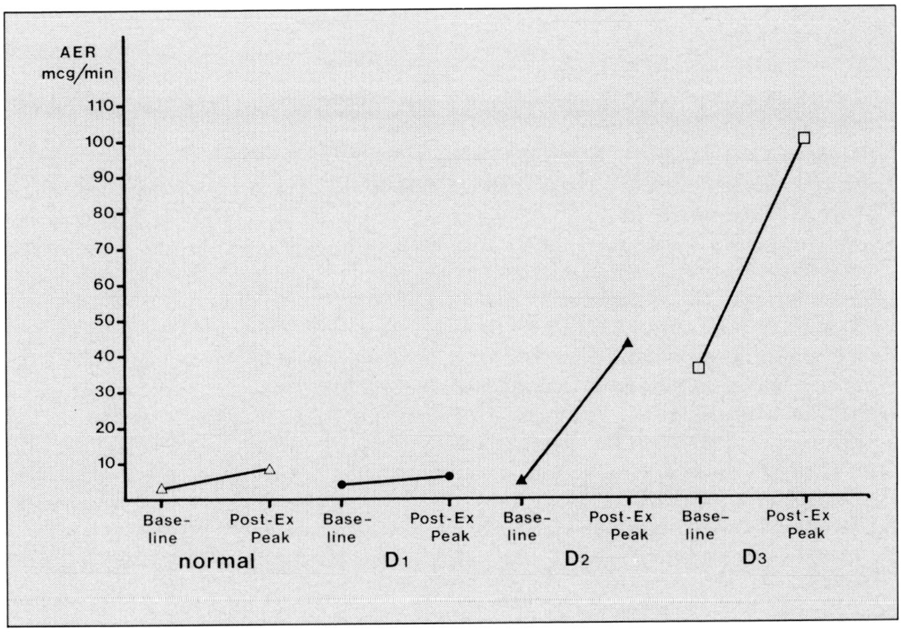

Fig. 5. Basal and postexcercise peak AER in 11 normal children and 87 type 1 diabetic children divided into three groups (D1–3). Group 1: 62 diabetic children with baseline and postexercise peak in the normal range. Group 2: 14 diabetic children with baseline AER in the normal range, but postexercise peak AER above the upper limit of normals. Group 3: 11 diabetic children with baseline AER above the upper limit of normals. HbA1 and duration of disease were significantly higher in groups 2 and 3 than in group 1.

Prevention and Therapy

No treatment is yet available to arrest the decline of kidney function in Albustix-positive diabetics. So new therapies to normalize the metabolic control in short-term diabetics are needed to prevent diabetic nephropathy as well as the other diabetic complications. However, such treatments are available only for short-term periods (artificial beta cell) or for limited trials (pancreas transplantation).

For the time being, the only possibility of preventing diabetic nephropathy lies in the early identification of the risk factors for its development during the course of diabetes. This is particularly important in diabetic children because in the first years of diabetes these factors can be easily modified [8, 59, 60]. It is thus useful to identify diabetic children with high GFR, kidney hypertrophy, basal microalbuminuria, or postexercise microalbuminuria. A large number of studies have shown that all the above renal abnormalities are normalized by strict metabolic control in the early stage of diabetes [8, 59, 60].

Antihypertensive therapy with beta blockers can slow the decline in kidney function of diabetic patients with diabetic nephropathy [1], and a reduction of AER in microalbuminuric diabetics has been observed [61]. However, this treatment, suggested for type 1 diabetic patients with microalbuminuria, but blood pressure still in the normal range, must be confirmed by long-term studies before it can be used extensively [61].

GFR can be lowered in normal man by a low-protein diet [62]. This approach was recently taken also in adult normoproteinuric hyperfiltering diabetics, bringing the raised GFR down to a near-normal level [63]. However, no similar studies are available to confirm these results in diabetic children.

In conclusion, strict metabolic control, antihypertensive treatment, and dietary protein restriction are the current means of controlling the risk factors for diabetic nephropathy observed in some long-term diabetics. Short-term correction of early diabetic renal abnormalities has been well documented, but the long-term efficacy of such treatment will be confirmed only over the next few years.

References

1 Parving, H.-H.; Andersen, A.R.; Smidt, U.M.; Sandahl Christiansen, J.; Oxenboll, B.; Svendsen, P.A.: Diabetic nephropathy and arterial hypertension. The effect of antihypertensive treatment. Diabetes *32:* suppl. 2, pp. 83–87 (1983).
2 Viberti, G.C.; Bilous, R.W.; Mackintosh, D.; Bending, J.J.; Keen, H.: Long-term correction of hyperglycaemia and progression of renal failure in insulin-dependent diabetes. Br. med. J. *286:* 598–602 (1983).
3 Andersen, A.R.; Sandahl Christiansen, J.; Andersen, J.K.; Kreiner, S.; Deckert, T.: Diabetic nephropathy in type 1 (insulin-dependent) diabetes: an epidemiological study. Diabetologia *25:* 496–501 (1983).
4 Knowles, H.C.: Magnitude of the renal failure problem in diabetic patients. Kidney int., suppl. 1, pp. 2–7 (1974).

5 Frokjaer Thomsen, O.; Andersen, A.R.; Sandahl Christiansen, J.; Deckert, T.: Renal changes in long-term type 1 (insulin-dependent) diabetic patients with and without clinical nephropathy: a light microscopic, morphometric study of autopsy material. Diabetologia *26:* 361–365 (1984).
6 Mogensen, C.E.: Kidney function and glomerular permeability to macromolecules in early juvenile diabetes. Scand. J. clin. Lab. Invest. *28:* 79–90 (1971).
7 Mogensen, C.E.; Christensen, C.K.; Vittinghus, E.: The stages in diabetic renal disease with emphasis on the stage of incipient diabetic nephropathy. Diabetes *32:* suppl. 2, pp. 64–78 (1983).
8 Mogensen, C.E.; Andersen, M.J.F.: Increased kindey size and glomerular filtration rate in untreated juvenile diabetes: normalization by insulin treatment. Diabetologia *11:* 221–224 (1975).
9 Sandahl Christiansen, J.; Frandsen, M.; Svendsen, P.A.; Gammelgaard, J.; Parving, H.-H.: Rapid changes in kidney function. Factors influencing kidney function in diabetic and normal man. Acta endocr., suppl. 242 (1981).
10 Mogensen, C.E.: Urinary albumin excretion in early and long-term juvenile diabetes. Scand. J. clin. Lab. Invest. *28:* 183–193 (1971).
11 Mogensen, C.E.: Pathophysiology of diabetic complications. Abnormal physiological processes in kidney; in Brownlee, Handbook of diabetes, vol. 4: Biochemical pathology, pp. 23–85 (STPM Press, New York 1981).
12 Osterby, R.; Gundersen, H.J.G.: Glomerular size and structure in diabetes mellitus. Diabetologia *11:* 225–229 (1975).
13 Osterby, R.: Early phases in the development of diabetic glomerulopathy. A quantitative electron microscopic study. Acta med. scand., suppl. 574 (1975).
14 Sandahl Christiansen, J.; Gammelgaard, J.; Frandsen, M.; Parving, H.-H.: Increased kidney size, glomerular filtration rate and renal plasma flow in short-term insulin-dependent diabetes. Diabetologia *20:* 451–456 (1981).
15 Wiseman, M.J.; Viberti, G.C.; Keen, H.: Threshold effect of plasma glucose in the glomerular hyperfiltration of diabetes. Nephron *38:* 257–260 (1984).
16 Mogensen, C.E.; Vittinghus, E.: Urinary albumin excretion during exercise in juvenile diabetes. Scand. J. clin. Lab. Invest. *35:* 295–300 (1975).
17 Huttunen, N.-P.; Kaar, M.-L.; Puukka, R.; Akerblom, H.K.: Exercise-induced proteinuria in children and adolescents with type 1 (insulin-dependent) diabetes. Diabetologia *21:* 495–497 (1981).
18 Osterby, R.; Gundersen, H.J.G.; Horlyck, A.; Kroustrup, J.P.; Nyberg, G.; Westberg, G.: Diabetic glomerulopathy. Structural characteristics of the early and advanced stages. Diabetes *32:* suppl. 2, pp. 79–82 (1983).
19 Osterby, R.; Andersen, A.R.; Gundersen, H.J.G.; Mogensen, C.E.; Parving, H.-H.: Quantitative studies of glomerular ultrastructure in juvenile diabetic patients with incipient nephropathy (Abstract). Diabetologia *27:* 317 (1984).
20 Viberti, G.C.; Bilous, R.W.; Mackintosh, D.; Keen, H.: Monitoring glomerular function in diabetic nephropathy. A prospective study. Am. J. Med. *74:* 256–263 (1983).
21 Kimmelstiel, P.: Diabetic nephropathy; in Becker, Structural basis of renal disease, p. 468 (Harper & Row, New York 1968).
22 Kroustrup, J.P.; Gundersen, H.J.G.; Osterby, R.: Glomerular size and structure in diabetes mellitus. Diabetologia *13:* 207–210 (1977).
23 Hostetter, T.H.; Troy, J.L.; Brenner, B.M.: Glomerular hemodynamics in experimental diabetes mellitus. Kidney int. *19:* 410–418 (1981).
24 Dizel, J.; Junker, K.: Abnormal glomerular filtration rate, renal plasma flow and renal protein excretion in recent and short-term diabetics. Br. med. J. *ii:* 13–19 (1972).
25 Mogensen, C.E.: Glomerular filtration rate and renal plasma flow in short-term and long-term juvenile diabetes mellitus. Scand. J. clin. Lab. Invest. *28:* 91–100 (1971).
26 Mogensen, C.E.: Renal function changes in diabetes. Diabetes *25:* 872–879 (1976).
27 Sandahl Christiansen, J.; Frandsen, M.; Parving, H.H.: Effect of intravenous glucose infusion on renal function in normal man and in insulin dependent diabetics. Diabetologia *21:* 368–373 (1981).
28 Sandahl Christiansen, J.; Frandsen, M.; Parving, H.-H.: The effect of intravenous insulin infusion on kidney function in insulin depedent diabetes mellitus. Diabetologia *20:* 199–204 (1981).
29 Parving, H.-H.; Noer, I.; Mogensen, C.E.; Svendsen, P.A.: Kidney function in normal man during short-term growth hormone infusion. Acta endocr. *89:* 796–800 (1978).
30 Parving, H.-H.; Sandahl Christiansen, J.; Noer, I.; Mogensen, C.E.: The effect of glucagon infusion on kidney function in short-term insulin-dependent juvenile diabetics. Diabetologia *19:* 350–354 (1980).
31 Wiseman, M.J.; Drury, P.L.; Keen, H.; Viberti, G.C.: Plasma renin activity in insulin-dependent diabetics with raised glomerular filtration rate. Clin. Endocr. *21:* 409–414 (1984).
32 Hostetter, T.H.; Olson, J.L.; Rennke, H.G.; Venkatachalam, M.A.; Brenner, B.M.: Hyperfiltration in remnant nephrons: a potentially adverse response to renal ablation. Am. J. Physiol. F *241:* 85–93 (1981).
33 Steffes, M.W.; Brown, D.M.; Maver, S.M.: Diabetic glomerulopathy following unilateral nephrectomy in the rat. Diabetes *27:* 35–41 (1978).
34 Elema, J.D.: Is one kidney sufficient? Kidney int. *9:* 308 (1976).
35 Brenner, B.M.; Hostetter, T.H.; Olson, J.L.; Rennke, H.G.; Venkatachalam, M.A.: The role of glomerular hyperfiltration in the initiation and progression of diabetic nephropathy. Acta endocr., suppl. 242, pp. 7–10 (1981).
36 Viberti, G.C.; Keen, H.: The patterns of proteinuria in diabetes mellitus. Diabetes *33:* 686–692 (1984).
37 Brenner, B.M.; Hostetter, T.H.; Humes, H.D.: Molecular basis of proteinuria of glomerular origin. New Engl. J. Med. *298:* 826–833 (1978).
38 Mogensen, C.E.; Solling, K.: Studies on renal tubular protein reabsorption: partial and near complete inhibition by certain amino acids. Scand. J. clin. Lab. Invest. *37:* 477–486 (1977).
39 Viberti, G.C.; Mackintosh, D.; Bilous, R.W.; Pickup, J.C.; Keen, H.: Proteinuria in diabetes mellitus: role of spontaneous and experimental variation of glycemia. Kidney int. *21:* 714–720 (1982).
40 Viberti, G.C.; Mackintosh, D.; Keen, H.: Determinants of the penetration of proteins through the glomerular barrier in insulin-dependent diabetes mellitus. Diabetes *32:* suppl. 2, pp. 92–95 (1983).
41 Parving, H.H.; Rutili, F.; Granath, K.; Noer, I.; Deckert, T.; Lyngsoe, J.; Lassen, N.A.: Effect of metabolic regulation on renal

leakiness to dextran molecules in short-term insulin-dependent diabetics. Diabetologia *17:* 157–160 (1979).
42 Viberti, G.C.; Pickup, J.C.; Jarrett, R.J.; Keen, H.: Effect of control of blood glucose on urinary excretion of albumin and β_2-microglobulin in insulin-dependent diabetes. New Engl. J. Med. *300:* 638–641 (1979).
43 Parthasarathy, N.; Spiro, R.G.: Effect of diabetes on glycosaminoglycan component of the human glomerular basement membrane. Diabetes *31:* 738–741 (1982).
44 Brownlee, M.; Spiro, R.G.: Glomerular basement membrane metabolism in the diabetic rat. Diabetes *28:* 121–125 (1979).
45 Ellis, D.; Becker, D.J.; Daneman, D.; Lobes, L.; Drash, A.L.: Proteinuria in children with insulin dependent diabetes: relationship to duration of disease metabolic control and retinal changes. J. Pediat. *102:* 673–680 (1983).
46 Poortmans, J.; Dorchy, H.; Toussaint, D.: Urinary excretion of total proteins, albumin, and β_2-microglobulin during rest and exercise in diabetic adolescents with and without retinopathy. Diabetes Care *5:* 617–623 (1982).
47 Mogensen, C.E.; Christensen, C.K.: Predicting diabetic nephropathy in insulin dependent patients. New Engl. J. Med. *311:* 89–93 (1984).
48 Viberti, G.C.; Jarrett, R.J.; Mahmud, U.; Hill, R.D.; Argyropoulos, A.; Keen, H.: Microalbuminuria as a predictor of clinical nephropathy in insulin-dependent diabetes mellitus. Lancet *i:* 1430–1432 (1982).
49 Price, D.A.; Fielding, B.A.; Davies, A.G.; Postlethwaite, R.J.: Short-term variability of urinary albumin excretion in normal and diabetic children. Diabetic Nephropathy *4:* 169–173 (1985).
50 Pravis, L.B.: Evaluation of clinical clues; in Rudolph, Pediatrics; 17th ed., p. 1165 (Appleton-Century Crofts, Norwalk 1982).
51 Rowe, D.J.F.; Bagga, H.; Betts, P.B.: Normal variations in rate of albumin excretion and albumin to creatinine ratios in overnight and daytime urine collections in non-diabetic children. Br. med. J. *291:* 693–694 (1985).
52 Rowe, D.J.F.; Hayward, M.; Bagga, H.; Betts, P.: Effect of glycaemic control and duration of disease on overnight albumin excretion in diabetic children. Br. med. J. *289:* 957–959 (1984).
53 Brouhard, B.; Allen, K.; Sapire, D.; Travis, L.B.: Effect of exercise on urinary N-acetyl-beta-*D*-glucosaminidase activity and albumin excretion in children with type I diabetes mellitus. Diabetes Care *8:* 466–472 (1985).
54 Hagstam, K.E.; Nordenfelt, I.; Svensson, L.; Svensson, S.E.: Comparison of different methods for determination of glomerular filtration rate in renal disease. Scand. J. clin. Lab. Invest. *34:* 31–36 (1974).
55 Dodge, W.F.; Travis, L.B.; Daeschner, C.W.: Comparison of endogenous creatinine clearance with inulin clearance. Am. J. Dis. Child. *113:* 683–692 (1967).
56 Cole, B.R.; Giangiacomo, J.; Ingelfinger, J.R.; Robson, A.M.: Measurement of renal function without urine collection. A critical evaluation of the constant infusion technic for determination of inulin and para-aminohippurate. New Engl. J. Med. *287:* 1109–1114 (1972).
57 Hricak, S.; Lieto, L.P.: Sonographic determination of renal volume. Radiology *148:* 311–312 (1983).
58 Wiseman, M.; Viberti, G.C.; Mackintosh, D.; Jarrett, R.J.; Keen, H.: Glycaemia, arterial pressure and micro-albuminuria in type 1 (insulin-dependent) diabetes mellitus. Diabetologia *26:* 401–405 (1984).
59 Viberti, G.C.; Pickup, J.C.; Bilous, R.W.; Keen, H.: Correction of exercise-induced microalbuminuria in insulin-dependent diabetics after 3 weeks of subcutaneous insulin infusion. Diabetes *30:* 818–823 (1981).
60 Wiseman, M.J., Saunders, A.J.; Keen, H.; Viberti, G.C.: Effect of blood glucose control on increased glomerular filtration rate and kidney size in insulin-dependent diabetes. New Engl. J. Med. *312:* 617–621 (1985).
61 Christensen, C.K.; Mogensen, C.E.: Reversal of progression in urinary albumin excretion in incipient diabetic nephropathy by antihypertensive treatment (Abstract). Diabetes Res. Clin. Pract., suppl. 1, p. 100 (1985).
62 Pullman, T.N.; Alvin, A.S.; Dern, R.J.; Landowne, M.: The influence of dietary protein on specific renal functions in normal man. J. Lab. clin. Med. *44:* 420–332 (1954).
63 Viberti, G.C.; Bognetti, E.; Wiseman, M.J.: Renal response to protein loading and modulating effect of plasma glucose in insulin-dependent diabetics with high and normal glomerular filtration rate (Abstract). XXIInd Congr. Eur. Dialysis Transplant Ass.-Eur. Renal Ass., Brussels 1985, p. 37.

Received: February 4, 1986

Giuseppe Chiumello,
Ospedale 'Luigi Sacco',
Clinica Pediatrica III°,
via G.B. Grassi 74,
I-20157 Milano (Italy)

Pediatrician *12:* 208–212 (1983–85)

0300–1245/85/0124–0208$2.75/0

Honeymoon Period in Insulin-Dependent Diabetes mellitus

E. Heinze, A. Thon

Department of Pediatrics, University of Ulm, FRG

Key Words. Remission · C-peptide · Immunosuppression · Islet growth

Abstract. The honeymoon period in type I diabetic patients is characterized by the preserved B cell function. Early diagnosis and rigorous insulin therapy at the time of diagnosis determine beginning and duration of postinitial remission. Age and sex, two other important variables for remission, cannot be influenced at all. Thus the possibility for a very young severely decompensated girl to experience a honeymoon period of long duration is significantly less compared to a teenage boy with moderately elevated blood glucose concentration at the time of diagnosis. Immunosuppression is currently under investigation to interrupt the ongoing self-destruction of the remaining B cells. The ultimate goal of therapy is to enhance islet cell growth.

Introduction

The remission phase in insulin-dependent diabetes mellitus (IDDM) may be characterized as the time after diagnosis when a good or excellent metabolic control is achieved with a low exogenous insulin requirement [1]. No generally accepted and concise definition for postinitial remission is available. However, for clinical use *Akerblom* [2] formulated a useful definition. He suggested that a patient has reached postinitial remission when he has no or minimal glucosuria, an insulin requirement of less than 0.5 U/kg/day and a serum C-peptide concentration of above 0.5 ng/ml. When looking closely at *Akerblom's* definition, it is apparent that the endogenous insulin secretion determines whether a diabetic child will experience a remission phase or not, which points to the morphology of the pancreas at or shortly after diagnosis.

The Pancreas

Gepts [3] and *Gepts and De Mey* [4] have contributed most to our knowledge on the pathology of IDDM, although *Opie* [5] in 1910 was the first to describe the round-cell invasion, now known as small lymphocytes, of the endocrine pancreas. Several reports [6–8] confirmed his initial observation. For the problem of the remission phase, the islets of Langerhans in patients with IDDM of less than 6 months' duration are of particular importance. Two obvious populations of islet tissue were examined. One group consisted of insulin-deficient islets which were shrunken but contained the normal number of glucagon-secreting A cells and somatostatin-secreting D cells [4]. The other group consisted of islets containing insulin-secreting B cells which were often hypertrophic. In one report [8] the number of islets in 2 untreated diabetics was the same as that in the control group. On average the number was reduced for all patients to one seventh of that of the controls. In another very recent report [9] attention was drawn to the fact that 9 diabetic children, who had had the disease for less than 6 months, all had insulin-containing islets in their pancreas, though in 2 of them the number was rather small. Nevertheless, in most patients with recent-onset diabetes mellitus the pancreas showed a considerable number of insulin-containing B cells. Thus from a morphological point of view it may be suspected that besides the anatomical changes a functional abnormality of the islets to secrete insulin may contribute to the manifestation of the disease.

C-Peptide Secretion

C-peptide and insulin are secreted in equimolar amounts from the B cells. 15 years ago radioimmunoassays for C-peptide were developed [10, 11]. Since that time C-peptide release in juvenile diabetic patients has been intensively studied. Before 1970 it was difficult to reliably measure endogenous insulin secretion in patients receiving exogenous insulin.

It soon became apparent that at the time of diagnosis fasting as well as stimulated C-peptide concentrations were low or completely non-existent.

At diagnosis *Block* et al. [12, 13] could not show any C-peptide release in response to an oral glucose challenge in ketoacidotic patients. After recovery, 2 weeks later, the same stimulus clearly augmented C-peptide release from the pancreas, though a delayed response was observed. The maximal C-peptide concentrations were reached after 2–3 h during the oral glucose tolerance test [13, 14]. In contrast to oral glucose, an intravenous glucose load did not stimulate C-peptide release, and different from healthy subjects [15], the priming effect of glucose on a second intravenous glucose challenge was completely abolished [16].

The infusion of arginine to type I diabetics during remission clearly stimulated C-peptide release, reaching the normal or lower normal range [14, 15, 17, 18]. Interestingly enough, similar to healthy subjects [19], an intravenous glucose tolerance test followed by an arginine infusion amplified the effect of the amino acid on C-peptide release [14]. The results indicate that during the remission of juvenile-onset diabetes the endocrine pancreas is selectively impaired and does not recognize glucose as an appropriate signal for C-peptide release but can transform the amplifying effect of glucose into a higher arginine-induced hormonal secretion rate.

It is largely unknown why the B cells do not respond to glucose by secreting insulin during remission. Recently, a 40,000-dalton glycoprotein was isolated from rat B cell membranes. An antibody raised against this protein completely blocked the glucose-induced insulin release from both rat islet and rat insulinoma cells [20]. If confirmed in man and by in vivo studies, the 40,000-dalton glycoprotein or similar proteins could explain the largely selective B cell defect during remission. In clinical practice the glucagon test is the most widespread stimulus to measure C-peptide release during remission. Initially the results of this test were compared to those measured after a standard breakfast. The responses of the endocrine pancreas to the meal and to glucagon were correlated, indicating a high predictive value of the glucagon test as to how the B cells will respond during normal daily life [21]. Patients with C-peptide concentrations exceeding 0.30 pmol/ml 6 min after an intravenous glucagon bolus were considered to be in remission [22]. Finally, the natural course of the residual B cell function during remission was prospectively studied. It was found that the highest stimulated C-peptide concentrations were measured 60–90 days after diagnosis and appropriate treatment [23]. During the subsequent months C-peptide secretion would decline as the B cell loss continued. At present the B cell destruction is thought to be the consequence of the ongoing immunological process, a topic presented by *Doberson* [50] in this volume.

Factors Determining Remission

The number of children who will experience a postinitial remission varies considerably from 6 to 100% [24–26]. During the last two decades a trend towards a higher frequency of remissions has been observed. Nowadays on average 30–80% of newly diagnosed diabetic children will ultimately enter the honeymoon period [18, 27–29]. The factors which contribute to the possibility of a remission in a diabetic child may be classified as metabolic and nonmetabolic. The nonmetabolic parameters, primarily age and sex, cannot be influenced at all. In several studies there was a significant correlation between the occurrence of a remission and age. These observations have been based on clinical criteria for a remission and also on the measurement of serum C-peptides or as 24-hour C-peptide excretion [17, 30, 31]. The possibility of younger children experiencing a remission is significantly smaller compared to older age groups. A sex difference for entering the honeymoon period has been reported. Boys are more likely to reach the remission period than girls [28, 31, 32]. As to the duration of remission in relation to sex, it was shown in one study that the honeymoon period was longest in older boys [28].

Initial treatment and the metabolic decompensation at the time of diagnosis seem to determine the frequency and the duration of remission. *Brush* [33] was the first to show that a rigorous insulin therapy at the beginning of the disease increased the frequency of subsequent remissions; this was confirmed by others [27, 32, 34]. In one study postinitial remission occurred in 39 out of 42 children (92%) admitted to one hospital and in 4 out of 16 children (25%) in another hospital [27]. This conspicuous difference in the occurrence of the remission between the two hospitals was related to a slower decrease in blood glucose at onset and a higher mean blood sugar concentration during the 1st week in the hospital with a low remission frequency. Prospectively it was possible to demonstrate that strict insulin therapy with nine daily injections increased C-peptide secretion during a test meal after 2 weeks by nearly 100% [34] when compared to a conventionally treated group of newly diagnosed diabetic patients.

Similarly to the frequency, the length of time before a patient enters remission depends primarily on the initial metabolic decompensation, which may be indicated by the hemoglobin A_{1C} (HbA_{1C} concentration at diagnosis. HbA_{1C} determined the time elapsed until an excellent metabolic control was achieved, defined as the day when all blood glucose determinations of the daily profile were and stayed below 150 mg/dl until discharge from hospital. Entry into remission occurred on day 4 or 5. This result was obtained in non-ketoacidotic patients with an insulin therapy of 1 U/kg/day of one third regular and two thirds NPH insulin. Two thirds of the daily insulin dose was given in the morning and one third in the evening [29, 35]. Patients, who quickly achieved good control, needed a lower insulin dose, which implies that they either had more endogenous insulin left or were more sensitive to exogenous insulin [29]. In a very recent report, it was concluded that clinical remission in type I diabetic patients may result both from the recovery of endogenous insulin secretion and from the enhancement of insulin sensitivity [36]. The lack of a concise definition of post-initial remission in IDDM hampers a comparison of its duration in different studies. Children seen in the Joslin Clinic between 1953 and 1958 had on average a duration of remission of 15 months [32]. In a Swedish study before 1973 the honeymoon period lasted 1.8 months [31]. In Finland, from 1964 to 1979, the mean duration of remission was 8.4 months, with the shortest period lasting 1 month and the longest 37 months [28]. In a recent combined study from Switzerland and Germany partial remission lasted 6.5 months with a standard deviation of 4.9 months [37].

The metabolic decompensation at diagnosis but not the initial insulin regimen contributes to the duration of remission. To evaluate the honeymoon period, stimulated serum C-peptide concentrations were determined. Patients who were initially treated with an intensified insulin regimen had a better secretory capacity after 2 weeks but not after 3 or 6 months, when compared to a conventionally treated group [34].

In contrast, the duration of the honeymoon period was found to correlate with the initial metabolic decompensation, represented by the HbA_{1C} concentration at diagnosis, the duration of glucosuria and the mean insulin requirement during the first 2 days of treatment [26, 38, 39].

It is of interest to note that HbA_{1C} correlated negatively with serum C-peptide, indicating that residual B cell function protected the diabetic child from severely decompensating [38, 40].

To summarize the influence of the metabolic factors on remission, the chain of events may be formulated as follows: an early diagnosis maintains a certain residual B cell function, prevents severe metabolic decompensation and increases the chance of the diabetic to quickly enter a long period of remission if a vigorous insulin treatment is initiated within the first few days.

Immunotherapy

Currently, immunotherapy of human autoimmune diseases such as type I diabetes mellitus means general immunosuppression. Most clinical immunologists would favor the specific deletion or suppression of autoreactive lymphocytes, particularly regulatory T lymphocytes with a specificity for autoantigen [41].

In IDDM many attempts to prolong the honeymoon period have been suggested or carried out. Small, mostly uncontrolled trials in which newly diagnosed type I diabetic patients have been immunosuppressed with corticosteroids, azathioprine, antilymphocyte immunoglobulin, levamisole and plasmapheresis have given inconclusive results [for a review see ref. 42].

At present cyclosporin A has attracted most attention for prolonging a remission. This drug is a potent inhibitor of T-helper-cell-dependent, cell-mediated and humoral immune response, and acts primarily at the level of T helper cells, probably by inhibiting lymphokine production [43].

In the two studies published so far, cyclosporin A induced and maintained the remission period. In 30 children and adolescents who received cyclosporin within 6 weeks of diagnosis insulin could be withdrawn in 20–50% for up to 285 days, indicating that they had reached a complete honeymoon period [44]. This event is normally observed in only 3% of diabetic patients [28]. Similar results were obtained in 12 recently diagnosed type I diabetics [24]. The two uncontrolled studies are, however, too short to draw any practical conclusions for the treatment of diabetic children. It appears that one has to weigh a possible benefit of a cyclosporin therapy against the sometimes serious side effects of the drug.

Conclusion and Outlook

The honeymoon period of type I diabetes mellitus is a challenge to indefinitely prolong its duration. With the currently available therapy 60–80% of patients will reach remission. Early diagnosis and vigorous insulin therapy at the manifestation of the disease mainly determine the beginning and duration of remission. These two variables can be controlled, while age and sex cannot be influenced at all. Thus a very young girl is significantly less likely to enter the honeymoon period than a teenage boy.

The residual B cell function of the endocrine pancreas determines whether a partial or a complete remission will be reached. Since type I diabetes mellitus appears to be an autoimmune process, numerous attempts have been made to prolong the honeymoon period by immunosuppression. At present, cyclosporin appears to be the most promising, but still investigative, drug to prolong remission.

The aim of immunotherapy is to interrupt the ongoing self-destruction of the insulin-producing B cells. For the future, it appears that research will be concentrated on stimulating the remaining B cells to divide and grow. Reports on human islet growth are scarce, but an increase in the number of islets up to 3 years of age and in their size up to 21 years of age has been noted [45].

Thus, the mitotic activity in adult islets seems to be low. Under the conditions of an increased demand for insulin, like pregnancy or obesity, an increase in the number of B cells takes place [for a review, see ref. 46]. Some animal studies, mostly on mice and rats, about islet cell growth should be briefly mentioned. From the steroid hormones, dehydroepiandrosterone metabolites but not cortisol, progesterone or estrogens stimulated B cell replication [47, for a review, see ref. 48].

Recently it has been shown that the insulin-like growth factor I was synthesized by the islets of Langerhaus. The synthesis was growth-hormone-independent. However, both growth hormone and insulin-like growth factor I augmented islet cell replication [48, 49].

At present many of the side effects of the above-mentioned hormones and our lack of knowledge of islet cell growth make it impossible to transform the results of animal studies into clinical trials to possibly prolong the honeymoon period of diabetic children.

References

1 Baker, L.; Kaye, R.; Root, A.W.: The early partial remission of juvenile diabetes mellitus. The roles of insulin and growth hormone. J. Pediat. *77:* 825–831 (1967).

2 Akerblom, H.K.: Definition of a partial remission in insulin-dependent, juvenile onset diabetes mellitus. Acta paediat. belg. *33:* 66–67 (1980).

3 Gepts, W.: Pathologic anatomy of the pancreas in juvenile diabetes mellitus. Diabetes *14:* 619–623 (1965).

4 Gepts, W.; De Mey, J.: Islet cell survival determined by morphology – an immunocytochemical study of the islets of Langerhans in juvenile diabetes mellitus. Diabetes *27:* suppl. 1, pp. 251–261 (1978).

5 Opie, E.L.: Disease of the pancreas (Lippincott, Philadelphia 1910).

6 MacLean, N., Ogilvie, R.F.: Observations on the pancreatic islet tissue of young diabetic subjects. Diabetes *8:* 83–91 (1959).

7 Junker, K.; Egberg, J.; Kromann, H.; Nerup, J.: An autopsy study of the islets of Langerhans in acute-onset juvenile diabetes mellitus. Acta pathol. microbiol. scand., A, Pathol. *85:* 699–706 (1977).

8 Doniach, J.; Morgan, A.G.: Islets of Langerhans in juvenile diabetes mellitus. Clin. Endocrinol. *2:* 233–248 (1973).

9 Foulis, A.K.; Stewart, I.A.: The pancreas in recent-onset type I (insulin-dependent) diabetes mellitus: insulin content of islets, insulitis and associated changes in the exocrine acinar tissue. Diabetologia *26:* 456–461 (1984).

10 Melani, F.; Rubenstein, A.H.; Oyer, P.E.; Steiner, D.F.: Identification of proinsulin and C-peptide in human serum by a specific immunoassay. Proc. natn. Acad. Sci. USA *67:* 148–155 (1970).

11 Beischer, W.; Keller, L.; Maas, M.; Schiefer, E.; Pfeiffer, E.F.: Human C-peptide. I. Radioimmunoassay. Klin. Wschr. *54:* 709–716 (1976).

12 Block, M.B.; Mako, M.E.; Steiner, D.F.; Rubenstein, A.H.: Diabetic ketoacidosis: evidence for C-peptide and proinsulin secretion following recovery. J. clin. Endocr. Metab. *35:* 402–406 (1972).

13 Block, M.B.; Rosenfield, R.L.; Mako, M.E.; Steiner, D.F.; Rubenstein, A.H.: Sequential changes in beta-cell function in insulin-treated diabetic patients assessed by C-peptide immunoreactivity. New Engl. J. Med. *288:* 1144–1148 (1973).

14 Vetter, U.; Heinze, E.; Thon, A.; Beischer, W.; Teller, W.M.: The effect of glucose, tolbutamide, and arginine on C-peptide release during remission in type I diabetes mellitus. Eur. J. Pediat. *140:* 305–310 (1983).

15 Koncz, L.; Soeldner, J.S.; Otto, H.; Smith, T.M.; Gleason, R.E.: Insulin secretory dynamics after two consecutive intravenous stimulations with glucose and/or tolbutamide. Metabolism *28:* 1183–1197 (1979).

16 Heinze, E.; Beischer, W.; Keller, L.; Winkler, G.; Teller, W.M.; Pfeiffer, E.F.: C-peptide secretion during the remission phase of juvenile diabetes. Diabetes *27:* 670–676 (1978).

17 Menchini, M.; Meschi, F.; Lambiax, R.; Puzzovia, M.; Del Guerico, M.J.; Chiumello, G.: C-peptide response to arginine stimulation in diabetic children. J. Pediat. *96:* 362–366 (1980).

18 Menzel, R.; Albrecht, G.; Jutzi, E.; Michaelis, D.; Ziegler, M.; Hildmann, W.: Remission phase in juvenile diabetes. Pathophysiology and influencing factors. Diabetologia *14:* 255 (1978).

19 Levin, S.R.; Karam, J.H.; Hane, S.; Grodsky, G.M.; Forsham,

P.H.: Enhancement of arginine-induced insulin secretion in man by prior administration of glucose. Diabetes *20:* 171–176 (1971).
20 Baekkeskov, S.; Lernmark, A.: A β-cell glycoprotein of M_r 40,000 is the major rat cell immunogen following xenogenic immunisation. Diabetologia *27:* 70–73 (1984).
21 Faber, O.K.; Binder, C.: C-peptide response to glucagon. A test for the residual β-cell function in diabetes mellitus. Diabetes *26:* 605–610 (1977).
22 Madsbad, S.; McNair, P.; Faber, O.K.; Binder, C.; Christiansen, C.; Transbol, J.: Beta-cell function and metabolic control in insulin treated diabetics. Acta endocr. *93:* 196–200 (1980).
23 Madsbad, S.; Krarup, T.; Regeur, L.; Faber, O.K.; Binder, C.: Insulin secretory reserve in insulin-dependent patients at time of diagnosis and the first 180 days of insulin treatment. Acta endocr. *95:* 359–363 (1980).
24 Assan, R.; Debray-Sachs, M.; Labovie, C.; Chatenoud, L.; Feutren, G.; Quiniou-Debrie, M.C.; Thomas, G.; Bachr, J.F.: Metabolic and immunological effects of cyclosporin in recently diagnosed type I diabetes mellitus. Lancet *i:* 67–71 (1985).
25 Mirouze, J.; Selam, J.L.; Pham, T.C.; Mendozu, E.; Ovsetti, A.: Sustained insulin-induced remission of juvenile diabetes by means of an external artificial pancreas. Diabetologia *14:* 223–227 (1978).
26 Vetter, U.; Heinze, E.; Beischer, W.; Kleihauer, E.; Teller, W.M.: Haemoglobin A_{1C}: a predictor for the duration of the remission phase in juvenile insulin-dependent diabetic patients. Acta paediat. scand. *69:* 481–483 (1980).
27 Ludvigsson, J.; Hägglöf, B.; Holmgren, G.: Early remission in juvenile diabetes. Excerpta Med. Int. Congr. Ser., No. 481, p. 145 (1979).
28 Knip, M.; Säkkinen, A.; Huttunen, N.P.; Käär, M.L.; Länkelä, A.; Mustonen, A.; Akerblom, H.K.: Postinitial remission in diabetic children – an analysis of 178 cases. Acta paediat. scand. *71:* 901–908 (1982).
29 Heinze, E.; Thon, A.; Vetter, U.: Initial metabolic decompensation and subsequent remission. Paediat. adolesc. Endocr. (in press).
30 Cosseley, J.R.; James, H.G.; Elliott, R.B.; Berrymann, L.C.; Edgar, B.W.: Residual beta-cell function and islet cell antibodies in diabetic children. Pediat. Res. *15:* 62–65 (1981).
31 Ludvigsson, J.; Heding, L.G.; Larsson, Y.; Leander, E.: C-peptide in juvenile diabetics beyond the postinitial remission period. Relation to clinical manifestations at onset, remission and diabetic control. Acta paediat. scand. *66:* 177–184 (1977).
32 White, P.; Graham, C.A.: The child with diabetes; in Marble, White, Bradley, Krall, Joslin's diabetes mellitus; 11th ed., pp. 339–360 (Lea & Febiger, Philadelphia 1971).
33 Brush, J.M.: Initial stabilization of the diabetic child. Am. J. Dis. Child. *67:* 429–444 (1944).
34 Madsbad, S.; Krarup, I.; Faber, O.K.; Binder, C.; Regeur, L.: The transient effect of strict glaecemic control on B-cell function in newly diagnosed type I (insulin-dependent) diabetic patients. Diabetologia *22:* 16–17 (1982).
35 Thon, A.; Heinze, E.; Vetter, U.; Teller, W.M.: Diabetes mellitus: Initialtherapie der Erstmanifestation mit Mischinsulin. Mschr. Kinderheilk. *132:* 803–806 (1984).
36 Yki-Järrinen, H.; Koivisto, V.A.: Insulin sensitivity in newly diagnosed type I diabetics after ketoacidosis and after three months of insulin therapy. J. clin. Endocr. Metab. *59:* 371–378 (1984).
37 Heinze, E.; Thon, A.; Vetter, U.; Gaedicke, G.; Zuppinger, K.: Gamma-globulin therapy in 6 newly diagnosed diabetic children. Acta paediat. scand. *74:* 605–606 (1985).
38 Knip, M.; Punkka, R.; Käär, M.L.; Akerblom, H.K.: Remission phase, endogenous insulin secretion and metabolic control in diabetic children. Acta diabet. lat. *19:* 243–251 (1982).
39 Vetter, U.; Heinze, E.; Kohne, E.; Teller, W.M.; Kleinauer, E.: Relation between the degree of initial decompensation and the duration of the remission phase in type I diabetes mellitus. Eur. J. Pediat. *138:* 63–66 (1982).
40 Heinze, E.; Kohne, E.; Meissner, C.; Beischer, W.; Teller, W.M.; Kleinhauer, E.: Hemoglobin A_{1C} (HbA_{1C}) in children with long standing and newly diagnosed diabetes mellitus. Acta paediat. scand. *68:* 609–612 (1979).
41 Kolb, H.; Toyka, K.V.: New concept in immunotherapy. Immunol. today *5:* 307–308 (1984).
42 Cahill, G.F.: Early intervention in insulin-dependent diabetes mellitus. Curr. Probl. clin. Biochem. *12:* 108–118 (1983).
43 Bendtzen, K.; Petersen, I.: Effect of cyclosporin A (CyA) on the immune response. CyA competitively inhibits the function of monocyte/macrophage-derived T-lymphocyte-activating factor. Immunol. Lett. *5:* 331–336 (1982).
44 Stiller, C.R.; Dupré, I.; Gent, M.; Jeaner, M.R.; Keown, P.A.; Lampacis, A.; Martell, R.; Rodger, N.W.; Graffenried, B.; Wolfe, B.M.I.: Effects of cyclosporin immunosuppression in insulin-dependent diabetes mellitus of recent onset. Science *223:* 1362–1367 (1984).
45 Ogilvie, R.F.: The endocrine pancreas in humans and experimental diabetes; in Cameron, O'Connor, The biology of diabetes mellitus and its complications. Ciba Fdn Coll. Endocr., vol. 15, pp. 49–66 (Churchill, London 1964).
46 Hellerström, C.: Growth pattern of pancreatic islets in animals; in Volk, Wellmann, The diabetic pancreas, pp. 61–97 (Plenum Press, New York 1977).
47 Coleman, D.L.; Leiter, E.H.; Applezweig, N.: Therapeutic effects of dehydroepiandrosterone metabolites in diabetes mutant mice (C 57 BL/KsJ-db/db). Endocrinology *115:* 239–243 (1984).
48 Nielsen, J.H.: Growth and function of the pancreatic β-cell in vitro. Acta endocr. *108:* suppl. 266, pp. 7–39 (1985).
49 Romanus, J.A.; Rabinovitch, A.; Rechler, M.M.: Neonatal rat islet cell cultures synthesize insulin-like growth factor I. Diabetes *34:* 696–702 (1985).
50 Duberson, M.: Pediatrician (1986).

Received: November 25, 1985

Eberhard Heinze, MD,
Department of Pediatrics,
University of Ulm,
Prittwitzstrasse 43,
D–7900 Ulm (FRG)

Pediatrician *12:* 213–219 (1983–85)

0300–1245/85/0124–0213$2.75/0

The Role of Trace Elements in Juvenile Diabetes mellitus

Torsten Tuvemo, Mehari Gebre-Medhin

Department of Pediatrics, University Hospital, Uppsala, Sweden

Key Words. Diabetes mellitus, insulin-dependent · Trace elements · Magnesium · Adolescents

Abstract. There is accumulating evidence that the metabolism of several trace elements is altered in insulin-dependent diabetes mellitus and that these nutrients might have specific roles in the pathogenesis and progress of this disease. Magnesium deficiency is the most evident disturbance of metal metabolism in diabetes mellitus. Hypomagnesemia might increase the risk of ischemic heart disease and severe retinopathy. Increased urinary loss of zinc is a commonly encountered feature of diabetes. High-dose oral zinc might enhance wound healing, although data regarding diabetes are lacking. Chromium increases tissue sensitivity to insulin and tends to raise high-density lipoprotein (HDL) cholesterol and the HDL:low-density lipoprotein ratio. Selenium is involved in processes which protect the cell against oxidative damage by peroxides produced from lipid metabolism. There is one report of elevated serum selenium in diabetic children although the clinical significance of this finding is still unclear. An insulin-like effect has recently been attributed to vanadium in experimental animals, a finding of potential interest to man. Current knowledge does not implicate iron, iodine, manganese, cobolt, nickel, silicone, fluoride, molybdenum or tin in the pathophysiology of diabetes. Appropriate trace element supplementation might prove beneficial in ameliorating some physiological deficiencies associated with diabetes and prevent or retard secondary complications. However, properly designed and well-documented trials, especially on magnesium supplementation, need to be performed before rationales for such supplementation are developed. The potential roles of vanadium, chromium and selenium in diabetes constitute challenging areas for further experimental and clinical research.

Introduction

Trace elements are those present in the body in concentrations of less than 0.01% of the total body weight. Currently, some 14 trace elements have been recognized to be of nutritional importance to mammals. These include iron, iodine, copper, zinc, manganese, cobalt, selenium, chromium, nickel, silicon, fluorine, vanadium, molybdenum, and tin. Other elements, normally considered as toxic such as arsenic, lead and cadmium, have a borderline effect on animal growth when excluded from experimental diets. Chromium, manganese, iron, cobalt, copper, zinc, selenium, molybdenum, and iodine are already recognized to be of physiological importance in man.

Many of these trace elements have at least one and, in many instances, many specific physiological roles. The biological functions of some of the trace elements have not yet been identified. Some of these trace elements are regarded essential in man because of their occurrence in certain nutrients, such as cobalt in vitamin B_{12}, or in certain enzymes such as molybdenum as a component of xanthine oxidase. The major recognized functions of trace elements relate to enzyme systems where they may act either as cofactors for metal-ion-activated enzymes or as specific constituents of metalloenzymes. Some other trace elements are constituents of proteins and hormones such as iodine in thyroxin and chromium as a cofactor for insulin. Thus, trace elements are apparently necessary for the normal function of several crucial metabolic pathways [1].

Deficiency of trace elements can arise from a primary cause such as low dietary intake or failure of intestinal absorption caused by an inborn error of metabolism. More commonly, they occur as a secondary consequence of organic disease, infectious illness and accidental or surgical trauma. Treatment with drugs, parenteral nutrition and hemodialysis can also induce trace element disorders. The signs and symptoms of trace element deficiency are corrected by either oral or intravenous therapy with the appropriate trace element.

There are several reasons for considering a role for trace elements in the pathogenesis and progress of insulin-dependent diabetes mellitus. Several trace elements have a role in tissue metabolism as antioxidants. Others, like chromium, influence glucose metabolism and tolerance [2–4]. Zinc restitution in diabetes mellitus may contribute to improved wound healing [5, 6] as well as improved T-lymphocyte function [7]. However, another side effect of zinc supplementation, namely reduced high-density lipoprotein (HDL) cholesterol in young healthy subjects may prove disadvantageous for subjects who have diabetes [8]. Hence trace elements may play an important role in ameliorating some physiological deficits associated with diabetes mellitus and prevent or retard dreaded secondary complications. In this review we will shortly summarize current knowledge on trace elements and magnesium relevant to insulin-dependent diabetes in young people.

Zinc

First thought to be mostly harmful, then of questionable importance, zinc is now known to be essential for the growth, development, and survival of all living matter [9]. Zinc is now identified as having an important role in zinc-containing metallo-enzymes, many of which play a fundamental role in critical enzymes in DNA, RNA and protein synthesis and degradation [10]. Despite being identified in more than 200 enzymes, many of the biological effects of zinc are still unexplained.

Zinc absorbtion from the bowel may be enhanced by a zinc-binding ligand. *Evans* [11] has suggested that this ligand is a tryptophan metabolite, picolinic acid, secreted from the exocrine pancreas. Many other compounds may also act as ligands that enhance zinc absorption. Approximately 20–30% of ingested dietary zinc is absorbed. High contents of calcium, phytate, fiber and chelating agents in the diet interfere with zinc absorbtion. Normal daily zinc intake in adults is approximately 12–15 mg. Urinary zinc loss is around 0.5 mg/day. A similar amount is lost by perspiration. Endogenous zinc loss in the gastrointestinal tract amounts to 1–2 mg/day.

Since 1934 when *Scott* [12] demonstrated that crystalline insulin contains considerable amounts of zinc, a great number of studies on the relation between zinc and diabetes have been performed. In many of these studies, zinc deficiency has been associated with reduced glucose tolerance [13], while in other studies no such difference could be shown [14, 15]. Zinc given intravenously has been shown to inhibit the diabetogenic effect of alloxane [16]. But this finding is of doubtful relevance for human diabetes.

Urinary losses of zinc seem to be increased in diabetic humans [17–20]. In the latter study on diabetic children and adolescents, 79 healthy controls excreted 3.2 ± 0.2 µmol/10 h while the diabetes group with 2 to 14 years duration of disease excreted 6.2 ± 0.5 µmol/10 h [20]. Renal zinc clearance was doubled in this group compared with controls. Also in recently diagnosed diabetics zinc clearance was significantly higher than in controls in that study [20].

Dietary intake of zinc in a group of diabetic children in Uppsala, Sweden, was about 40% higher than in matched healthy controls [21]. In streptozotocin-induced diabetes in rats, recent studies have demonstrated increased intestinal uptake of zinc from the food [22] and accumulation of zinc in liver and kidney [23].

The reports on zinc concentrations in serum, erythrocytes and tissues have given contradictory results. Both decreased, normal and high serum and plasma zinc levels have been reported [e.g. 24, 25]. *Hägglöf* et al. [20] found decreased serum zinc concentrations during the first days after the onset of diabetes. This was normalized after 1 month but, in diabetics with 2 to 14 years duration serum zinc was slightly lower than in controls. The zinc content in hair from diabetic children and adolescents did not differ from that in controls. In our material we found no difference between diabetic children and controls regarding serum zinc levels [26]. In a family study involving 30 families with a diabetic child and 30 control families, serum zinc did not differ between the diabetic children and controls. There was also no difference between the diabetic relatives and controls [*Hägglöf*, personal commun.]. In this study a sex difference was obvious with low serum zinc in diabetic females but relatively high serum zinc in diabetic males. If this is true it might explain some of the controversies in earlier reports.

It seems that diabetics have a clearly increased urine excretion of zinc, but that this loss can probably be compensated for by an increased dietary intake or an increased utilization of dietary zinc. Whether the increased urinary excretion is secondary to a primarily too high intake or utilization or whether the increased utilization is a response to urinary loss is not clear from current, somewhat controversial data.

Impaired wound healing is a common late complication in at least older diabetics. Several studies have reported improved wound healing in non-diabetic patients following administration of high-dose oral zinc [27]. No such data are available for diabetics.

Copper

Copper is a component of several metallo-enzymes that are required for oxidative metabolism. These enzyme systems include cytochrome oxidase, ferroxidases, aminooxidases, superoxide dismutase, ascorbic acid oxidase, and tyrosinase. Cytochrome oxidase is a key enzyme for the production of most of the energy of metabolism in aerobic cells.

Ceruloplasmin accounts for more than 95% of the copper present in the blood plasma. It now appears that in addition to having a major role in copper transport, ceruloplasmin has an important ferroxidase activity. In this capacity it is necessary for the optimal rate of oxidation of Fe^{2+} from body stores in the liver and bone marrow to Fe^{3+}. This is a necessary step before iron can attach to transferrin for transport to and uptake by the erythrocyte precursors in the bone marrow.

Nutritional copper deficiency has only rarely been recognized in otherwise healthy, well-nourished infants and children. Copper deficiency has generally been described in premature infants, infants with multi-nutritional deficiency problems, during prolonged intravenous feeding, severe malabsorption and inherited metabolic disease. Since diabetic children consume a diet with a slightly higher protein content than non-diabetic children [21] and since their diet has a good representation of seafood and green vegetables, copper deficiency is unlikely to occur in juvenile diabetes mellitus with good dietary regimen.

Copper uptake from the intestinal lumen is increased three times in streptozotocin-induced diabetic rats. Therefore these animals accumulate copper in the tissue stores [22]. In a study on middle-aged human diabetics, *Noto* et al. [28] found higher copper levels in the diabetic patients than in controls, especially in the elderly diabetics. The authors suggest that hypercupremia might enhance the development of large vessel disease in diabetic humans. In childhood it seems from our data that copper levels, at least in serum, if increased are only marginally so [26]. In this age group this slight hypercupremia is probably not of clinical relevance. The slight increase in serum copper in diabetic children might be a reflection of a minor but not significant increase in ceruloplasmin observed in this disease [29].

Selenium

Human selenium intake varies with the source of the food and with food processing and cooking. The selenium content of food is related to the food's protein content and geographical origin [30]. Thus, animal meat, sea food, and unrefined cereal products are good sources of selenium, whereas refined carbohydrates, fruit, and vegetables are low in selenium content. The chemical form of selenium varies greatly and can affect its availability from diets and hence its biological action. Values for selenium in blood vary with the patient's country of origin and increase with age. Infants on special or restricted diets or with certain metabolic disorders have been found to have lower selenium levels than healthy children of the same age living in the same area.

Selenium is an integral part of the enzyme glutathione peroxidase, which is thought to interact with vitamin E in protecting the cell membrane against oxidative damage by peroxides produced from lipid metabolism [31]. A fall in selenium levels is usually accompanied by a corresponding fall in glutathione peroxidase. Whereas laboratory tests may suggest a state of selenium deficiency, clinical evidence for selenium deficiency is more equivocal. There are a few reported cases of muscle pain and tenderness resulting in an inability to walk in patients with low levels of serum selenium [32]. This condition responded to selenium supplementation alone within 1 week. Growth responses to selenite supplementation have also been recorded in children suffering from protein-energy malnutrition who had previously failed to respond to dietary treatment [33]. An endemic cardiomyopathy known as Keshan disease has been described in China and is associated with selenium deficiency [34].

In a recent report on young diabetics and healthy controls under our care [35], we found that the mean serum selenium concentration in the diabetic children, determined by neutron activation analysis, was significantly higher than in healthy controls. Boys and girls in both groups had nearly identical mean serum selenium levels and we found no correlation between the selenium concentrations and either the age, weight or height of the children and the indicators of diabetic control. This difference between our diabetic and healthy children was further validated by comparison of the mean for our controls with the mean found in a larger control population in our area.

Although the diabetic children under our care were consuming a diet with a slightly higher protein content than their healthy peers, we could not explain the elevated serum selenium levels in our diabetic subjects by protein intake alone. Since dietary protein is the most important source of selenium, serum selenium concentration was compared with protein intake [36]. A slight correlation was observed between serum selenium concentration and protein intake expressed as percent of the recommendations but this trend was not statistically significant.

In search of another explanation for the elevated serum selenium levels observed in our subjects we investigated alterations in the serum levels of selected metal transport proteins [36]. However, a comparison of serum selenium and selected serum proteins did not reveal any significant correlation except for prealbumin. Hence the generally elevated level of serum selenium in diabetic children cannot be explained by the diet intake or protein status described in our observations. We have suggested that our findings regarding selenium might be a response to some other metabolic abnormality or derangement in diabetes mellitus. In this context it is tempting to postulate that the elevated serum selenium in diabetic children might be a reponse to altered metabolism in this disease and that diabetics might have higher selenium needs than the general population.

Manganese

The nutritional importance of manganese in mammals has been recognized for many years, and there is substantial information on the effects of experimental manganese deficiency, the physiological role, and the metabolism of this element [37]. Yet, surprisingly little is known about human manganese status. It has been suggested that this is probably partly accounted for by the lack of established laboratory indicator of manganese status. There is only one report of human manganese deficiency, an adult person fed an experimental diet accidentally deficient in this nutrient [38]. Features of manganese deficiency include depressed vitamin-K-dependent clotting factors and a mild dermatitis.

Recent animal experiments suggest that in insulin deficiency, manganese enhances pancreatic protein synthesis in diabetic rats via a Ca^{++}-dependent mechanism [39]. The relevance of these findings for human diabetes is unknown.

Molybdenum

There has only been 1 case of acquired molybdenum deficiency described in humans [40]. In addition, there is a case report of a child who had demonstrated abnormalities of xanthine oxidase and sulfide oxidase, both of which contain molybdenum [41]. It was concluded that this child had an abnormality of molybdenum metabolism. In diabetes experience regarding this element is completely lacking.

Chromium

It is only recently that a physiological role for chromium was first suspected. The one well-documented role for chromium is as a cofactor for insulin. It is believed that chromium facilitates the initial attachment of insulin to peripheral insulin receptor sites [42]. The percentage of ingested chromium that is absorbed is largely dependent upon the chemical form of this element. Absorbtion of inorganic chromium is negligible (less than 1%) and its biological activity is small in comparison with that of a naturally occurring organic chromium complex that has been termed 'glucose tolerance factor' (GTF). The absorbtion of GTF chromium is at least 10% and possibly much higher. A substantial percentage of absorbed GTF chromium is detectable in the liver. It is thought that chromium is released into the circulation in response to an increase in circulating endogenous insulin and that this chromium facilitates the action of insulin at peripheral sites. The kidneys provide the major excretary root for this cation. It has also been postulated that excessive consumption of readily absorbable carbohydrates may contribute to chromium depletion by causing excessive urinary chromium excretion [43].

Chromium deficiency has been found only in cases of generalized protein-energy malnutrition among population groups with poor diet in some areas in the world and during total parenteral nutrition without added chromium [44]. The impaired glucose tolerance of these malnourished infants improved significantly after a single oral dose of 250 μg Cr^{3+} [45, 46]. It has also been shown that the weight gain of chromium-supplemented infants was significantly greater than that of control children.

Excessive chromium excretion, which has been observed in juvenile onset diabetics [47], may lead to chromium depletion [48]. High-chromium yeast supplementation has been reported to enhance tissue sensitivity to insulin in overt diabetics [49]. A similar supplementation in healthy subjects also tends to raise plasma levels of HDL cholesterol and the HDL/low-density lipoprotein ratio [50]. If confirmed, such an effect would be particularly valuable in many diabetics, in whom decreased HDL levels may contribute to an elevated risk of atherosclerotic disease.

Vanadium

The trace element vanadium has an unclear biological function. Reports from experimental work suggest that vanadate, an oxidized form of vanadium, appears to have an insulin-like action [51]. Female Wistar rats with streptozotocin-induced diabetes normalized their blood glucose levels during treatment with vanadate. In chicks, vanadium deficiency increases both plasma cholesterol and triglyceride levels [52, 53]. In humans no data seem to have been published on vanadium in diabetes.

Magnesium

Magnesium is a major mineral component of the human intracellular fluid and a constituent of bones and teeth. It comprises 0.5 g/kg human body weight, and is thus not defined as a trace element. It has important functions in the transmission of nerve impulses and muscle contraction, and acts as an activator and coenzyme in carbohydrate and protein metabolism and is also involved in the metabolism of potassium and calcium in humans. Deficiency states are characterized by neuromuscular dysfunction, convulsions, delirium, personality changes, and cardiac arythmia or arrest. Magnesium is absorbed in the ileum and primarily excreted in the urine. Its absorbtion is affected by total intake, intestinal transit time, rate of water absorbtion and the resulting intraluminal magnesium concentration in the ileum, and finally also by calcium, phosphate and lactose content in the diet. The absorbtion can be inhibited by high concentrations of phytic acid in the food. Foods with the highest content of magnesium are whole grains, dry beans, peas, soy beans, and nuts.

In 1978, *McNair* et al. [54] showed that adult diabetics are hypomagnesemic. Since then it has been shown that both pregnant and nonpregnant adult diabetics demonstrate lower serum magnesium levels than healthy controls [55, 56]. In a group of 27 children and adolescents, 5–18 years of age and with 2–15 years of diabetes, we found a mean serum magnesium level that was 10% below the mean for a control group [26]. Only 4 of the 27 diabetic children had values above the mean for healthy controls, while one third of the diabetics demonstrated serum magnesium values of 20 μg/ml or less (range for the normal controls 20–27 μg/ml). We also studied the nutrient density in the diet of 14 of these diabetic children and the healthy controls [21]. The mean magnesium content of the normal diet was 30 mg/1,000 kJ, while in the diabetic diet it was 39 mg/1,000 kJ. As the diabetic children had a mean energy intake that was 10–15% higher than the controls, the mean daily magnesium intake for the diabetic group was 40–50% higher than for the controls. The reason for hypomagnesemia in the diabetic children was, therefore, not a low intake. It has been shown that during glucosuria magnesium excretion in the urine is increased [57]. The reason for the hypomagnesemia in diabetics is probably mainly urinary losses [17]. Some residual endogenous insulin production does not protect against hypomagnesemia [58]. The degree of hypomagnesemia seems to be related to the duration of the disease. In adult diabetics it has been shown that the magnesium depots in trabecular bone and muscle are reduced [57, 59].

It has been suggested that hypomagnesemia increases the risk of ischemic heart disease [60]. It has also been reported that diabetics with severe retinopathy have lower serum magnesium levels than diabetics without obvious microvascular disorder [54], which has suggested a role of hypomagnesemia in the development of diabetic microangiopathy. Administration of magnesium has been shown to be protective against ischemic heart disease in animals with experimental magnesium dificiency [60]. It seems likely that magnesium deficiency may play a role in the long-term complications of diabetes mellitus, and that supplementation may prove potentially beneficial. However, further studies are needed before decisions can be made on general magnesium supplementation in all diabetic patients.

References

1 Underwood, E.J.: Trace elements in human and animal nutrition (Academic Press, New York 1971).

2 Mertz, W.: Effects and metabolism of glucose tolerance factor. Nutr. Rev. *33:* 129–135 (1975).

3 Frieberg, J.M.; Schneider, T.R.; Streeten, D.H.; Schneider, A.J.: Effects of brewer's yeast on glucose tolerance. Diabetes *24:* 433 (1975).

4 Offenbacher, E.G.; Pi Sunyer, F.X.: Beneficial effect of chromium-rich yeast on glucose tolerance and blood lipids in elderly subjects. Diabetes *29:* 919–925 (1980).

5 Pories, W.S.; Henzel, J.H.; Rob, C.G.; Strain, W.H.: Acceleration of wound healing in man with zinc sulphate given by month. Lancet *i:* 121–124 (1967).

6 Cohen, C.: Zinc sulphate and bed sores. Br. med. J. *ii:* 561 (1968).

7 Duchateau, J.; Delessene, G.; Vrijens, R.; Collet, H.; Beneficial effects of oral zinc supplementation on the immune response of old people. Am. J. Med. *70:* 1001–1004 (1981).

8 Hooper, P.L.; Visconti, L.; Garry, P.J.; Johnson, G.E.: Zinc lowers high-density lipoprotein-cholesterol levels. J. Am. med. Ass. *244:* 1960–1961 (1980).

9 Vallee, B.L.; Wacker, W.E.C.: in Fasman, Handbook of biochemistry; 3rd ed., vol. II (CRC Press, Cleveland 1976).

10 Vallee, B.L.; Falchuk, K.H.: Zinc and gene expression. Phil. Trans. R. Soc. *294:* 185–197 (1981).

11 Evans, G.W.: Picolinic acid and zinc absorption; in Sarkar, Biological aspects of metals and metal-related diseases (Raven Press, New York 1983).

12 Scott, D.A.: Crystalline insulin. Biochem. J. *28:* 1592–1602 (1934).

13 Roth, H.P.; Kirchgessner, M.: Insulingehalte in Serum bzw. Plasma von Zinkmangelratten vor und nach Glucosestimulierung. Int. J. Vitam. Nutr. Res. *45:* 202–208 (1975).

14 Macapinbe, M.P.; Pearson, W.N.; Darby, W.J.: Some characteristics of zinc deficiency in the albius rat; in Prasad, Zinc metabolism (Thomas, Springfield 1966).

15 Quaterman, J.; Florence, E.: Observations on glucose tolerance and plasma levels of free fatty acids and insulin in the zinc-deficient rat. Br. J. Nutr. *29:* 75–79 (1972).

16 Awadallah, R.; Tahani, H.M.; El-Dessonkey, E.A.: Serum mineral changes due to exogenous ATP and certain trace elements in experimental diabetes. Z. Ernähr.Wiss. *18:* 1–7 (1979).

17 Tarmi, S.: Studies on zinc metabolism. III. Effects of the diabetic state on zinc metabolism. A clinical aspect. Endocr. Jap. *10:* 9–15 (1963).

18 Pidduck, H.G.; Wren, P.S.S.; Evans, O.A.: Plasma, zinc and copper in diabetes mellitus. Diabetes *19:* 234–239 (1970).

19 Canfield, W.K.; Hambidge, K.M.; Johnson, L.K.: Zinc nutriture in type I diabetes mellitus: relationship to growth measure and metabolic control. J. Pediat. Gastroent. Nutr. *3:* 577–584 (1984).

20 Hägglöf, B.; Hallmans, G.; Holmgren, G.; Ludvigsson, J.; Falkmer, S.: Prospective and retrospective studies of zinc concentrations in serum, blood clots, hair and urine in young patients with insulin-dependent diabetes mellitus. Acta endocr. scand. *102:* 88–95 (1983).

21 Kylberg, E.; Ewald, U.; Tuvemo, T.; Gebre-Medhin, M.: Dietary intake in Swedish diabetic children. Acta paediat. scand. *320:* 32–37 (1985).

22 Craft, N.E.; Failla, M.L.: Zinc, iron and copper absorption in the streptozotocin-diabetic rat. Am. J. Physiol. *244:* 122–128 (1983).

23 Failla, M.L.; Craft, N.; Weinberg, G.A.: Depressed response of plasma iron and zinc to endotoxin and GEM in STZ-diabetic rat. Proc. Soc. exp. Biol. Med. *172:* 445–448 (1983).

24 Martin, M.C.; Bustamente, J.; Fernandez, J.; Ortiz, O.: A study of the metabolism of zinc and its metallo-enzymes in diabetes mellitus. Biomedicine *23:* 134–136 (1975).

25 Melzer, J.E.; Rutman, J.; George, P.; Rutman, R.; Kitchell, J.R.: The urinary excretion pattern of trace metals in diabetes mellitus. Am. J. med. Sci. *244:* 282–289 (1962).

26 Ewald, U.; Gebre-Medhin, M.; Tuvemo, T.: Hypomagnesemia in diabetic children. Acta paediat. scand. *72:* 367–371 (1983).

27 Hallbook, T., Lanner, E.: Serum zinc and healing of chronic leg ulcers. Lancet *ii:* 780 (1972).

28 Noto, R.; Alicata, R.; Sfogliano, L.; Neri, S.; Bifarella, M.: A study of cupremia in a group of elderly diabetics. Acta diabet. lat. *20:* 81–85 (1983).

29 Gebre-Medhin, M.; Ewald, U.; Tuvemo, T.: Reduced serum proteins in diabetic children on a twice daily insulin schedule. Acta paediat. Scand. *74:* 961–965 (1985).

30 Scott, M.C.; Thompson, J.N.: Selenium content of feedstuffs and effects of dietary selenium levels upon tissue selenium in checks and poults. Poultry Sci. *50:* 1742–1748 (1971).

31 Tappel, S.C.: Selenium-glutathione peroxidase and vitamin E. Am. J. clin. Nutr. *27:* 960–965 (1974).

32 Van Rij, A.M.; Thomson, C.D.; McKenzie, J.M.; Robinson, M.F.: Selenium deficiency in total parenteral nutrition. Am. J. clin. Nutr. *32:* 2076–2085 (1979).

33 Schwartz, K.: Development and status of experimental work on factor 3 – selenium. Fed. Proc. *20:* 666–675 (1961).

34 Xiaoshu, C.; Xuecun C.; Gaunggui, Y.; et al.: Relation of selenium deficiency to the occurence of Keshan disease; in Spallholz, Martin, Ganther, Selenium in biology and medicine, pp. 171–175 (AVI Publishing, Westport 1981).

35 Gebre-Medhin, M.; Ewald, U.; Plantin, L.O.; Tuvemo, T.: Elevated serum selenium in diabetic children. Acta paediat. scand. *73:* 109–114 (1984).

36 Gebre-Medhin, M.; Kylberg, E.; Ewald, U.; Tuvemo, T.: Dietary intake, trace elements and serum protein status in young diabetics. Acta paediat. Scand. *320:* 38–43 (1985).

37 Leach, R.M.: in Prasad, Oberlas, Trace elements in human health and disease, vol.II (Academic Press, New York 1976).

38 Doisy, R.J.; Streeten, D.H.; Freiberg, J.M.; Schneider, A.S.: in Hemphill, Trace substances in environmental health, vol. VI (University of Missouri Press, Columbia 1972).

39 Korc, M.: Manganese action on protein synthesis in diabetic rat pancreas: evidence for a possible physiological role. J. Nutr. *114:* 2119–2126 (1984).

40 Abumrad, N.N.; Schneider, D.R.; Rogers, L.S.: Aquired molybdenum deficiency. Clin. Res. *27:* 774A (1979).

41 Duran, M.; Beemer, F.A.; Heiden, C.V.D.; Korteland, J.; de Bree, P.K.; Brink, M.; et al.: Combined deficiency of xanthine oxidase and sulphite oxidase: a defect of molybdenum metabolism or transport? J. inherit. metab. Dis. *1:* 175–178 (1978).

42 Christian, G.D.; Knoblock, E.C.; Purdy, W.C.; Mertz, W.: A polarographic study of chromium-insulin-mitochondrial interaction. Biochim. biophys. Acta *66:* 420–423 (1963).

43 Schroeder, H.A.: The role of chromium in mammalian nutrition. Am. J. clin. Nutr. *21:* 230–244 (1969).

44 Wallack, S.: Clinical and biochemical aspects of chromium deficiency. Am. Coll. Nutr. *4:* 107–120 (1985).
45 Gurson, C.T.; Saner, G.: Effect of chromium on glucose utilization in marasmic protein-calorie malnutrition. Am. J. clin. Nutr. *24:* 1313–1319 (1971).
46 Hopkins, L.L.; Ransome-Kuti, O.; Majaj, A.S.: Improvement of impaired carbohydrate metabolism by chromium 3 in malnourished infants. Am. J. clin. Nutr. *21:* 203–211 (1968).
47 Hambidge, K.M.: in Mertz, Cornatzer, New trace elements in nutrition, pp. 169–194 (Dekker, New York 1971).
48 Hambidge, K.M.: Chromium nutrition in man. Am. J. clin. Nutr. *27:* 505–514 (1974).
49 Elias, A.N.; Grossman, M.K.; Valenta, L.J.: Use of the artificial beta cell (ABC) in the assessment of periferal insulin sensitivity: effect of chromium supplementation in diabetes. Gen. Pharmacol. *15:* 535–539 (1984).
50 Elwood, J.C.; Nash, D.T.; Streeten, H.P.: Effect of high-chromium brewer's yeast on human serum lipids. J. Am. Coll. Nutr. *1:* 263–274 (1982).
51 Heyliger, C.E.; Tahihani, A.G.; McNeill, J.H.: Effect of vanadate on elevated blood glucose and dispersed cardiac performance of diabetic rats. Science *227:* 1474–1477 (1985).
52 Nielsen, F.H.: Newer trace elements, and possible application in man; in Prasad, Trace elements in human health and disease, vol. II (Academic Press, New York 1976).
53 Hopkins, L.L., Jr.; Mohr, H.E.: Vanadium as an essential nutrient. Fed. Proc. *33:* 1773–1775 (1974).
54 McNair, P.; Christiansen, C.; Madsbad, S.; et al.: Hypomagnesemia, a risk factor in diabetic retinopathy. Diabetes *27:* 1075–1077 (1978).
55 Matter, H.M.; Nisbet, J.A.; Burton, G.S.; et al.: Hypomagnesemia in diabetes. Clinica chim. Acta *95:* 235–242 (1979).
56 Mather, H.M.; Levin, G.E.: Magnesium state in diabetes. Lancet *i:* 924 (1979).
57 Johansson, G.; Danielsson, B.G.; Ljunghall, S.; Wibell, L.: Evidence for a disturbed magnesium metabolism in diabetes mellitus. Magnesium Bull. *3:* 178–180 (1982).
58 Menzel, R.; Pusch, H.; Ratzmann, G.W.; et al.: Serum magnesium in insulin-dependent diabetics and healthy subjects in relation to insulin secretion and glycemia during glucose-glucagon test. Exp. clin. Endocr. *85:* 81–88 (1985).
59 De Leeuw, I.; Vertommen, J.; Abs, R.: The magnesium content of the trabecular bone in diabetic subjects. Biomedicine *29:* 16–17 (1979).
60 Seelig, M.S.; Heggtveit, H.A.: Magnesium interrelationships in ischaemic heart disease: a review. Am. J. clin. Nutr. *27:* 59–79 (1974).

Received: January 30, 1986

Torsten Tuverno,
Department of Pediatrics,
University Hospital,
S-751 85 Uppsala (Sweden)

Pediatrician *12:* 220–228 (1983–85)

0300–1245/85/0124–0220$2.75/0

The Use of Insulin Pump Therapy in Adolescents[1]

Georgeanna J. Klingensmith, Beverly P. Giordano, Edward R. McCabe, Jessica J. Radcliffe

Children's Hospital, and Department of Pediatrics, University of Colorado School of Medicine, Denver, Colo., USA

Key Words. Diabetes · Glycohemoglobin · Continuous subcutaneous insulin infusion · Retinopathy · Nephropathy · Neuropathy · Home blood glucose monitoring

Abstract. Continuous subcutaneous insulin infusion (CSII) systems have been used in diabetes management since the mid-1970s. Investigators have reported encouraging results with CSII use in adult subjects with dramatically improved glucose control, reversal of some complications, and high acceptance and compliance rates. We have studied 10 adolescents and 3 young adults using CSII for diabetes management. Only the three young adults (ages 20, 24, 34 years) have had markedly improved metabolic control, sustained pump use, and made adequate psychological adjustment to CSII therapy. Adolescent subjects, (ages 9–17 years), experienced problems with peer acceptance of pumps, had difficulty with infusion needle insertion and skin care, were unable to perform home blood glucose monitoring consistently, made nonadvised manipulations of insulin dosage and reported mechanical problems with CSII devices more frequently than the young adult subjects. Mean duration of CSII use in adolescent subjects (6.1 months) was significantly less than mean use (30.6 months) among the young adults ($p < 0.01$). Currently, adults appear to have greater success than adolescents in using CSII for diabetes management.

Introduction

Diabetes mellitus has been recognized for centuries as a wasting illness accompanied by a profuse flow of sweet urine. Treatment in this early era was limited to dietary restrictions and enchantments. The discovery of insulin in 1921 was hailed as a cure for this previously fatal disorder, and administration of multiple daily doses of solubilized (regular) insulin did markedly improve the quality of life and life expectancy in young people with diabetes. During the 1940s it became apparent that long-term survival was frequently associated with development of microvascular disease resulting in poor peripheral circulation, blindness and renal failure.

A debate ensued over whether these microvascular complications are the result of abnormal glucose metabolism or were unrelated, but genetically closely associated, phenomena [1]. This debate cannot be resolved completely until we have the ability to normalize glucose metabolism in diabetic subjects. Only recently we have begun to develop management tools which may achieve this aim. Subcutaneous pumped insulin delivery is one of these tools which is anticipated to allow us to determine whether normalization of glucose metabolism can prevent microvascular disease.

Through the 1970s conventional treatment of diabetes mellitus consisted of a mixture of short and intermediate-acting insulin given once or twice a day, a meal plan restricting concentrated sugars and saturated fats, as well as daily urine tests for glucose and ketones. Exercise was encouraged as healthful, and home blood glucose monitoring was suggested for some selected young adults [2]. With this treatment plan the mean glycosylated hemoglo-

[1] Supported in part by the Clinical Research Center grant No. RR-69 from the General Clinical Research Centers Program of the Division of Research Resources, National Institutes of Health.

1
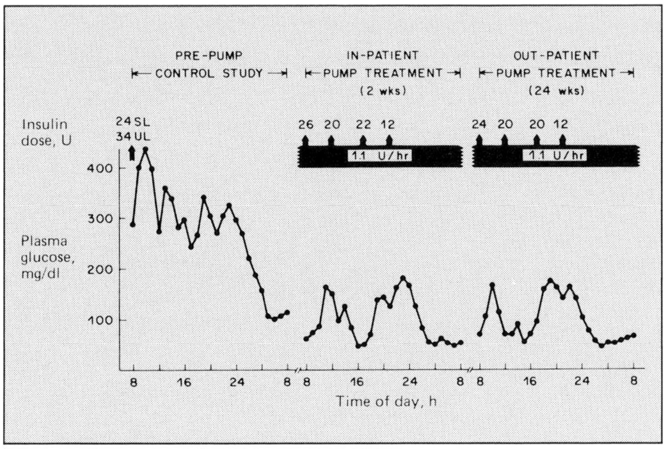

2
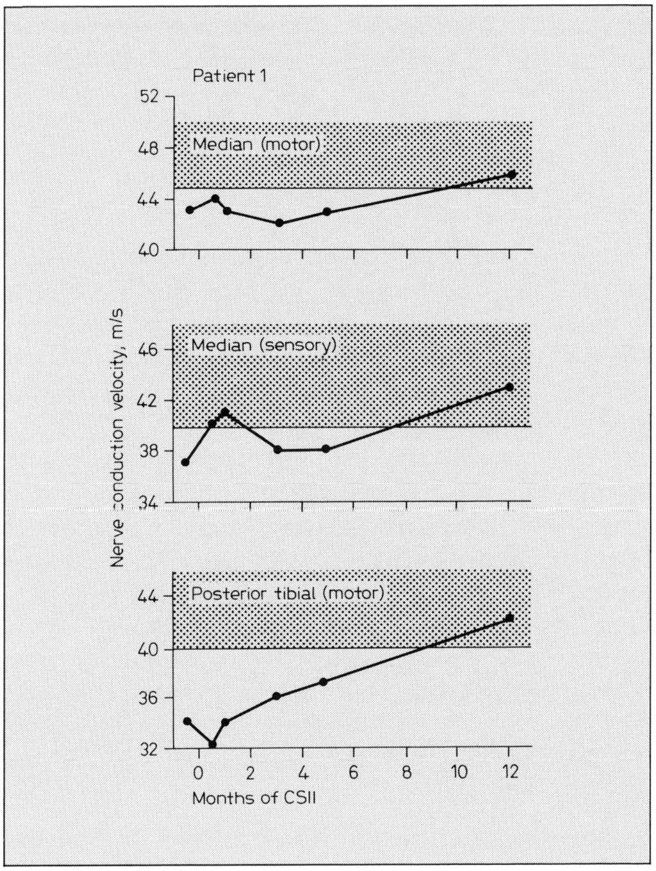

Fig. 1. Plasma glucose levels in a patient during conventional treatment at termination of a 2-week period of inpatient treatment with the infusion pump, and on readmission to the Clinical Research Center after 24 weeks of outpatient treatment with the infusion pump. The solid arrow at the upper left indicates insulin administration by conventional means. The stippled arrows indicate preprandial insulin doses delivered by the infusion pump in the doses shown. The number within the stippled bar indicates the basal rate of insulin delivery during treatment with infusion pump. SL = Semilente insulin; UL = ultralente insulin. Reprinted by permission from *Tamborlane* et al. [14].

Fig. 2. Nerve conduction velocity data on 1 patient before and during 1 year of CSII. Shaded areas represent normal values for each nerve tested. Reprinted by permision from *White* et al. [16].

bin level reported for pediatric patients was 150–180% of the upper limits of normal, suggesting that this form of conventional therapy did not achieve optimal blood glucose regulation [3–6].

As the evidence accumulates that the short-term metabolic abnormalities can be corrected with normalization of blood glucose, more emphasis has been placed on lowering daily blood glucose levels. Current management recommendations include daily blood glucose determinations, tailoring meal planning, insulin and exercise to daily blood glucose values, and consideration of multiple daily insulin injections [7]. The knowledge which makes these recommendations possible comes from experience with subcutaneous pumped insulin infusion systems.

In 1978 *Pickup* et al. [8] reported the normalization of blood glucose during short-term pumped insulin delivery in 12 adult subjects. The following year, *Tamborlane* et al. [9] also reported reduction to normal of plasma glucose in seven adolescents using a pumped subcutaneous insulin for a brief inpatient study period [9]. These infusion systems are nonglucose-regulated open-loop systems. Thus, the insulin dose administered is manually adjusted as indicated by intermittent peripheral glucose determinations.

Rapid publications followed which documented normalization of intermediary metabolites [10], catecholamine and growth hormone responses to exercise [11] and glucagon secretion [12] during treatment with portable insulin infusion pumps. Both *Pickup* et al. [13] and *Tamborlane* et al. [14] demonstrated the safety and efficacy of long-term outpatient treatment with insulin pumps (fig. 1).

Prolonged outpatient treatment with insulin infusion pumps has allowed assessment of improved glucose homeostasis on the complications associated with longstanding diabetes. Improvement in nerve conduction velocity (fig. 2), autonomic neuropathy, and a decrease in painful neuropathy have been found within 6 weeks of institution of insulin infusion pump therapy [15, 16]. An increase in growth velocity has been noted in some children and adolescents treated with insulin infusion pumps [16, 17].

An increase in capillary permeability may be one of the earliest lesions of the microvascular complications of diabetes. A decrease in exercise-induced glomerular capillary leakage of albumin after 2 weeks of insulin pump use was reported by *Koivisto* et al. [18] (fig. 3). *White* et al. [19] from St. Louis have found a return to normal in vitreous fluorescein leakage in subjects who normalize their glycohemoglobin during intensive therapy (fig. 4) [19]. Despite these encouraging reports of reversal of the initial lesion of microvascular disease, no change in the progression of nephropathy has been noted, and little improvement in established retinopathy has been found [20–23] (fig. 5). However, there is some hope that progression of retinopathy may be halted after 2–3 years of near-normal glycemia [24].

The equivocal or slight improvement in the long-standing complications of diabetes focused attention on longer-term studies using pumped insulin infusions to improve glucose regulation. Although occasional children and adolescents have been studied for 6 months or longer, most reports have been of adult subjects.

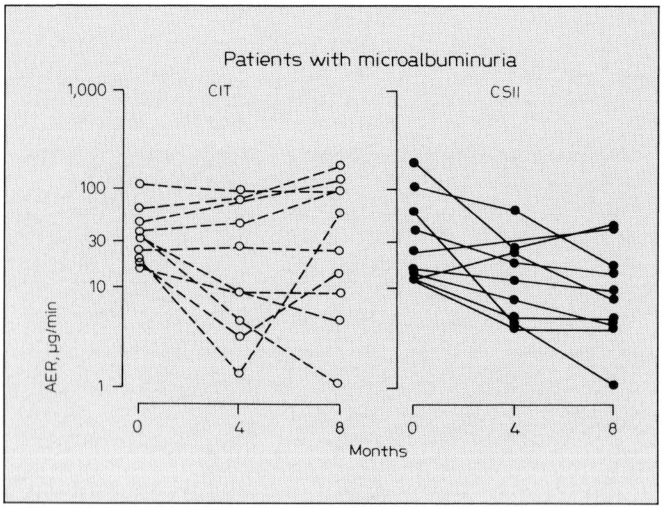

Fig. 3. Change in albumin excretion rate (AER) in 10 patients with baseline albumin excretion rates exceeding 12 mg/min. CIT = Conventional injection treatment. Reprinted by permission from the Kroc study [23].

Materials and Methods

Subjects

At the Children's Hospital, Denver, Colo., USA, and the University of Colorado Health Sciences Center, we studied the efficacy of continuous subcutaneous insulin infusion (CSII) in 13 children, adolescents and young adults. Patients selected for the pump protocol had an age range of 9–31 years at the initiation of pump therapy (table I). Three of the subjects were young adults with a mean age of 23.6 years (range 18–31 years). The mean age of the adolescent group was 13.6 years (range 9–17 years). In the young adult group the mean duration of diabetes was 15 years (range 4–26 years); the mean duration in the adolescent group was 6 years (range 1–13 years). Prior to entering the pump study, eight of the patients had been followed in the pediatric diabetes clinics at either the Children's Hospital, Denver, or the University of Colorado Health Sciences Center. The other 5 subjects were referred specifically for consideration of pump therapy.

Table I. CSII patient characteristics

		Age years	Duration of diabetes years	Duration of CSII therapy months
Young adults (n = 3)	mean	23.6	15	30.6*
	range	18–31	4–26	27–36
Adolescents (n = 10)	mean	13.6	6	6.1*
	range	9–17	1–13	0.1–16

* $p < 0.01$.

Indications

The indications for pumped insulin therapy included retinopathy (3), nephropathy (2), frequent hospitalizations for ketoacidosis (4), failure of conventional therapy (4), quest for optimal control (3), parental pressure (3), insulin management during steroid therapy for iritis (1), and desire to increase growth rate (1). Failure of conventional therapy was defined as the presence of two of the following three parameters: (1) glycosylated hemoglobin over 15% for 6–12 months, (2) fasting triglycerides greater than 3 times normal and (3) persistent ketonuria over a 6-month period.

Inpatient Study Design

Subjects were admitted to the Pediatric Clinic Research Center at the University of Colorado Health Sciences Center to initiate pump treatment. Prepump control data were collected for 2–3 days, while patients administered their usual intermittent subcutaneous insulin. They followed an American Diabetes/Dietetic Association exchange meal plan designed to provide 50–60 kcal/kg/day, with 80% of the calories contained in 3 meals and the remaining 20% divided between 2 snacks each day. Exercise at designated times using a stationary bicycle was encouraged throughout the hospitalization. Metabolic measurements in the prepump period included blood glucose determinations every 2 h; fasting cholesterol, triglycerides and free fatty acids; a glycosylated hemoglobin level; determinations of growth hormone, glucagon and amino acid values and a 24-hour urine collection for creatinine clearance, glucose and protein excretion.

The diabetes team psychologist and/or the clinical nurse specialist met with each patient and family during the prepump study

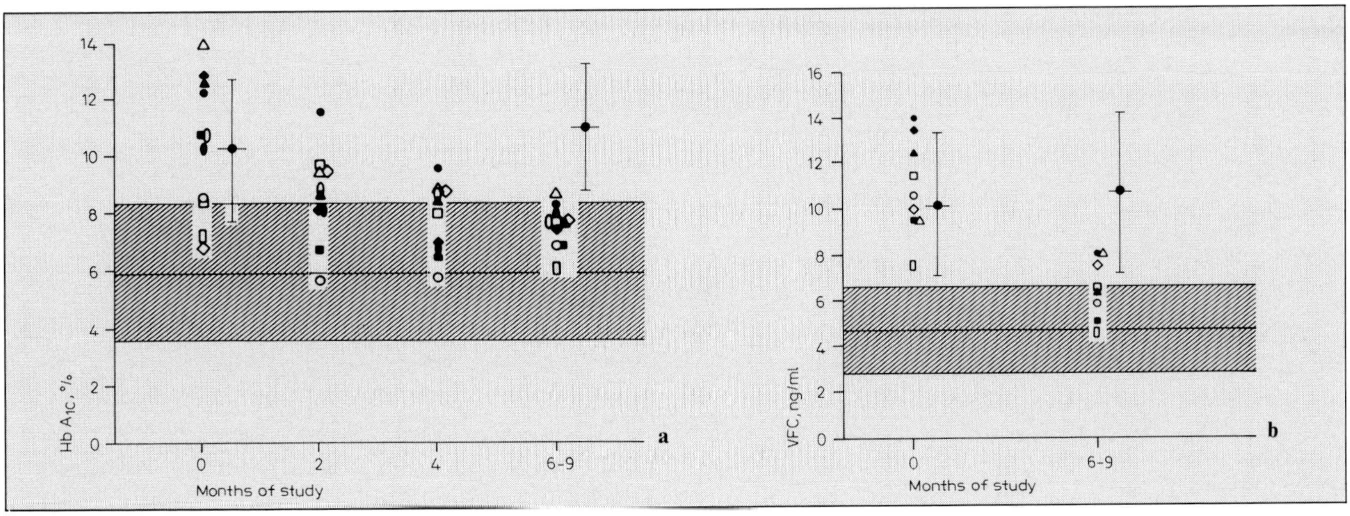

Fig. 4. Symbols fot 11 individual study subjects are the same in both panels. The bars represent the mean ± 1 SD for 25 conventionally treated diabetic subjects. The shaded area represents the mean ± 2 SD for nondiabetic controls. Reprinted by permission from *White* et al. [19]. **a** Hemoglobin A_{1C} in 11 subjects at initiation and after 2, 4, and 6–9 months of intensive insulin therapy. The reduction in hemoglobin A_{1C} in the intensively treated group over 6–9 months was significant ($p < 0.001$). **b** Fluorescein concentration in the posterior vitreous (VFC) of the 8 subjects from **a** with proliferative retinopathy and with stable orno background retinopathy 1 h after the intravenous injection of 7 mg/kg of fluorescein. Results are shown before and after 6–9 months of intensive therapy. The reduction in VFC in the intensively treated subjects was significant ($p < 0.001$).

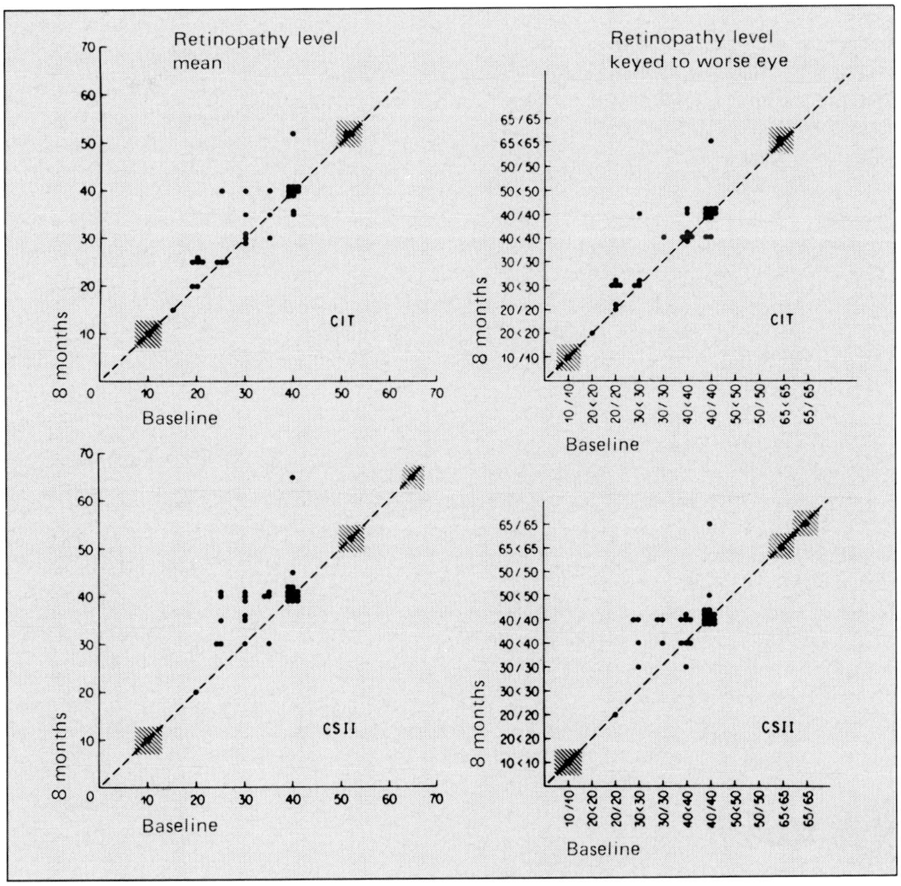

Fig. 5. Retinopathy levels at baseline and at 8 months in individual patients assigned to CSII or conventional injection treatment (CIT). There is no difference between the two groups. Values falling on the broken identity line indicate no change, those falling to the left of the line indicate deterioration, and those falling to the right indicate improvement. Retinopathy levels in patients initially selected for the trial but not meeting the eligibility criteria with respect to retinopathy are denoted by the shaded areas. Reprinted by permission from the Kroc study [23].

Table II. Glycohemoglobin (%) changes in first 6 months of CSII

		Baseline	1–2 months	6 months
Adults	mean	13.3	10.7	9.2
	range	10.0–17.6	8.2–12.2	7.6–12.4
	n	3	3	3
Adolescents	mean	15.2	14.1	14.5
	range	8.6–19.5	9.8–16.9	12.9–15.4
	n	10	7	3

Table III. Reasons given by adolescent patients for discontinuation of CSII therapy

Too much effort and attention required	7
Psychological discomfort, peer teasing	6
Inability to fully participate in athletics	5
Size of pump	4
Skin infections or tenderness	3
Decreased motivation	2

period to review their expectations of pumped insulin therapy, their understanding of the open-loop nature of the infusion system, and their ability to follow the pump protocol requirements. The nursing staff of the Clinical Research Center taught patients and families how to operate the pump, dilute the insulin and insert the infusion needle into the subcutaneous tissue. If patients were not already monitoring capillary blood glucose, this skill was introduced in the prepump period.

The total daily prepump insulin dose was used as the initial 24-hour insulin infusion dose. Initially, 50% of the dose was administered as the basal dose and 50% was divided into premeal bolus doses. Adjustments were made in the basal and bolus insulin infusion rates over the ensuing 2–10 days to achieve blood glucose values between 100 and 200 mg/dl.

Outpatient Study Design

Following discharge from the hospital, patients were instructed to maintain weekly telephone contact with the nurse specialist and were scheduled for monthly visits for the duration of the study. They were asked to test and record blood or urine glucose values several times each day, follow individualized meal plans, exercise daily, change the infusion needle every 1 to 2 days, and to administer the insulin doses as prescribed. All patients initially used the Auto Syringe 2-C infusion pump which measures 6.4 × 18.4 × 7.2 cm and weighs 480 gms. Three patients later used the smaller Auto Syringe 6-C pump that measures 8.3 × 15.8 × 2.5 cm and weighs 270 gms. The Auto Syringe 2-C pump has an exposed infusion syringe as well as exposed dials and infusion buttons. The 6-C model is encased and fits into a leather belt pack.

At each monthly visit glycohemoglobin, blood glucose and fasting cholesterol and triglycerides were measured. The physician, nurse specialist, and psychologist reviewed with each patient and family the adjustment of the infusion rate according to the blood glucose tests, the details of pump and needle site care and discussion of psychologic impact of using an infusion pump. Dietary changes were made as necessary.

Results

Glycohemoglobin

All 13 patients experienced short-term improvement in metabolic control as measured by decreased glycohemoglobin levels in the initial 1–2 months of pump therapy. Baseline glycohemoglobin values were elevated in all 13 patients. The mean baseline glycohemoglobin was 14.6% with a range of 8.6–19.5% (normal = 6.3–8.2%). The three young adult subjects began pump use with a mean glycosylated hemoglobin of 13.3%; after 2 months of pump therapy this value fell to 10.7% and was 9.2% at the end of 6 months of pumped insulin therapy. The 10 adolescents had a mean glycohemoglobin value of 15.2% at initiation of pump therapy. This was not significantly different from the young adults. Seven adolescents were still using pumps at the end of 2 months, and their mean glycohemoglobin was 14.1%. After 6 months, only 3 adolescents continued pump use; their mean glycohemoglobin was 14.6%. The adolescent values at 2 months and at 6 months were greater than the young adult values at these times (table II).

Duration of Use

Six years later, two of the three young adult patients continue to use pumped insulin therapy; both have purchased small sophisticated pumping devices. Mean duration of pump use in the ten adolescent subjects was 6.1 months, but median duration of pump use was only 2.5 months. None of these subjects use infusion systems at this time. The difference between duration of pump use between the young adults and the adolescent subjects is significant ($p < 0.01$).

The adolescent patients gave the reasons listed in table III for discontinuing pumped insulin therapy.

Growth

Despite the short-term use in our adolescent subjects, 3 did use pump therapy long enough to determine changes in growth rate. One mid-pubertal adolescent male had a growth rate of 3 cm per year for the year preceding pump therapy. During the 4 months of pump treatment he grew 7 cm, a rate of 21 cm/year. In the subsequent 9 months off pump therapy his growth rate decreased to 5.4 cm/year. A second trial of infusion therapy was undertaken with no change in growth rate. Throughout the initial 4-month treatment period, his glycohemoglobin remained below 10.5. During the second 10 month treatment period, his glycohemoglobin ranged from 14.6 to 17.2. The other two subjects had mild increases in their growth rates during the study period; however, these changes were not significantly different from the pre- or poststudy periods.

Microvascular Disease

The study was not designed to evaluate the effect of infusion therapy on microvascular complications of diabetes; however, several subjects had evidence of microvascular disease at the initiation of the study. One young adult had bilateral proliferative retinopathy prior to the study. He had stabilization of his retinopathy although he did require continued laser therapy for the initial 3 months of CSII treatment. Only a single treatment has been necessary in the subsequent 6 years. A second young adult developed proliferative retinopathy during infusion therapy. She suffered a retinal hemorrhage 18 months after initiation of infusion treatment. During that 18-month period, her mean glycosylated hemoglobin level was 13.9%. Following photocoagulation therapy, she became a motivated pump user, and her glycosylated hemoglobin values since have been less than 10.0%. No further laser therapy has been necessary.

Two of the young adults remained on pump therapy for at least 3 years and have had diabetes mellitus for longer than 15 years. One has been asymptomatic with normal blood pressure but has had a slowly falling creatinine clearance from 97 ml/min/1.73 m^2 to 50 ml/min/1.73 m^2, despite glycohemoglobin values of 5–6.9% (normal 5–7.9%). The other subject initiated infusion therapy when hypertension suggested diabetic nephropathy. Her creatinine clearance initially improved from 75.5 ml/min/1.73 m^2 to 115.9 ml/min/1.73 m^2 with normalization of her blood pressure. Over the subsequent year her creatinine clearance gradually fell to 70 ml/min/1.73 m^2 and has remained stable at this level for 3 years.

Discussion

Successful use of insulin pumps for 6–12 months have been reported in a few adolescent subjects. Successful use of pumped subcutaneous insulin therapy in 6 toddlers over a 6-month period has even been reported. During this 6-month study, glycosylated hemoglobin values decreased significantly and hypoglycemic episodes decreased both in frequency and severity for the toddlers [25].

Our experience in adolescent subjects is not as successful. Our adolescents were unable to adhere to the more rigorous demands in management placed on them and disliked the constant physical presence of the insulin pump and the subcutaneous needle. Other investigators also have been disenchanted with insulin infusion therapy in adolescents. *Stewart* et al. [26] of the Joslin Clinic treated 24 youngsters with insulin pumps for an average of 12 months (range 2–37 months). Thirty percent of their subjects discontinued pump therapy. The females in their study discontinued pump treatment because of the amount of work involved, weight gain, depression or continued poor control. Males discontinued pump use because of severe hypoglycemia or infusion site infection. Normalization of blood glucose and glycohemoglobin were not achieved. Noncompliance to the demands of a meal plan and self blood glucose monitoring continued to be a problem. The Joslin group concluded that more intense, frequent supervision might be needed if normalization of blood glucose was the goal of pumped insulin therapy in adolescents.

A survey of 53 pediatric diabetologists [27] found that only 7% viewed CSII as the treatment of choice for children and adolescents. The diabetologists surveyed treated an estimated 12,350 youngsters with diabetes and reported only 2.7% of their patients were using insulin pumps.

Complications associated with the insulin pumps also have dampened patient and physician interest. *Peden* et al. [28] reported an increased risk of diabetic ketoacidosis among the users of pumped insulin therapy. In 101 patients using insulin pumps, they reported 36 episodes of ketoacidosis in 1,880 patient months of pumped use. Forty-two percent of the episodes were thought to be related to problems unique to pumped insulin therapy. Since only regular insulin is administered, if the infusion is interrupted unwittingly, rapid insulin deficiency resulting in ketoacidosis may occur.

In 1984, a survey of the mortality among diabetic patients using CSII systems was reported [29]. Pumped insulin therapy was found to be associated with 35 known deaths. Two of these deaths were felt to be related directly to pump use. One 42-year-old male's death was attributed to hypoglycemia secondary to malfunction of the pumping device, and a 60-year-old female died of acute bacterial endocarditis, secondary to an abscess at the

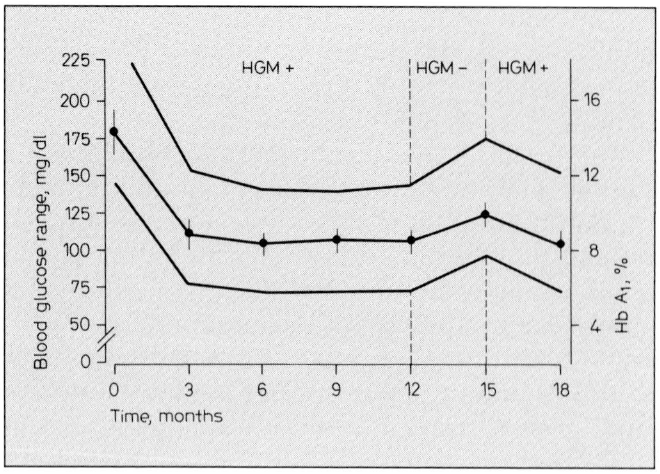

Fig. 6. Blood glucose range and mean hemoglobin A_1 obtained in patients given either CSII or multiple daily insulin doses. HGM+ depicts home monitoring of blood glucose 4 or more times each day. HGM– depicts monitoring 2 or fewer times each day.

catheter insertion site. Despite these two deaths, the Center for Disease Control investigators concluded that 35 deaths in an estimated 3,500 pump users in the United States was not greater than the expected number of deaths calculated from age-specific death rates for conventionally treated individuals with type I diabetes. The report did point out that users of pumped insulin therapy face a number of risks unique to this treatment modality, i.e., pump slowing causing hyperglycemia and ketoacidosis, pump runaway causing hypoglycemia, and catheter-induced infection. Investigators suggested that practitioners use stricter criteria in selecting patients for pumped insulin therapy. Patients with advanced nephropathy and neuropathy may be at greater risk for pump complications. Evaluation of patient motivation and compliance as well as recommendation of individualized realistic glycemic goals for each patient on pump therapy were also suggested. Improved pumps have been developed over the past 4 years which have variable pre-programmable rates as well as automatic shutdown and audible alarms for pump malfunction. These newer pumps may decrease the risk of pump-related ketoacidosis and hypoglycemia.

A report by *White* et al. [30] suggests that short-term testing with insulin infusion may identify candidates for intensive insulin therapy who have poor ability to recover spontaneously from hypoglycemia. Elimination of these subjects may reduce the risk of hypoglycemia with pumped insulin therapy.

The risk and expense associated with pumped insulin delivery has led to attempts to determine what components of infusion therapy have resulted in more normal glycemia. *Schriffin and Belmonte* [31] studied 21 patients using both insulin infusion pumps and intensive conventional therapy consisting of multiple daily subcutaneous insulin injections coupled with frequent self blood glucose monitoring and the use of algorithms to adjust insulin dose and food intake. The variable in this study associated with significant changes in glycohemoglobin levels was the frequency of blood glucose monitoring. Regardless of the method of insulin delivery, subjects who monitored blood glucose 4 times daily and made adjustments according to blood glucose values had significantly better glucose control than those who monitored less often (fig. 6). This study strongly suggests that a motivated, educated patient frequently can achieve near normal blood glucose using intensive conventional therapy.

Our experience with CSII in adolescents suggests that many adolescents are unsuccessful in using this mode of therapy. If current trends documenting the relationship between normalization of blood glucose metabolism and prevention of long-term sequelae of diabetes prove correct, then we must strive for normal or near normal blood glucose in our adolescent subjects. The insulin infusion pump may be one tool which we can use to achieve this, but appropriate patient selection is important.

What criteria should be used to select candidates for pumped insulin therapy? We recommend that pump therapy be considered only in individuals who have been unable to achieve the desired degree of glucose control with conventional or intensive conventional therapy. However, we do support the 1985 American Diabetes Association policy statement [32] that the choice also rests with the informed patient. Professionals supervising patients using insulin pumps should be experienced in insulin pump treatment and be prepared to offer 24-hour availability to pump users. Patients must be strongly motivated to improve glucose control and must be willing to assume substantial responsibility for their daily care. They should be able to demonstrate use of the insulin pump, perform self monitoring of blood glucose on a regular basis, and use the data so obtained to alter the insulin infusion rate. Patients should be taught the potential complications peculiar to pump therapy. We would strongly recommend that a psychologist be involved in the screening of potential adolescent pump candidates in order to aid in the assessment of the candidate's goals for pump therapy, his or her support systems and to evaluate the candidate's emotional stability. Parents desiring pumped insulin therapy for young children must understand the degree of work involved and should allow the youngster to wear a pump and infusion set for several days before making a decision about its use. Adolescents and their parents should clearly define their expectations of pumped insulin therapy as well as agree upon division of responsibilities related to using the insulin infusion pump.

Children whose parents are willing to monitor blood glucose levels regularly and make alterations in insulin, food and exercise may achieve improved metabolic control with pump therapy, providing the children can tolerate the inconvenience of the pump during exercise and other daily routines. Young adolescents may not desire or receive intensive parental involvement in their diabetes management and may be unable to carry out the daily tasks needed for successful pump use. Body image and self identity struggles in early adolescent years may also make pump use an unpopular choice. Since older adolescents and young adults are more future-oriented, they appear to be better candidates for insulin pump therapy. Prepregnancy metabolic control, desire to retard the development of microangiopathy, and flexibility in life style may be goals associated with pump use in this group.

For the average child or adolescent with diabetes, we would recommend a management program consisting of insulin given 2 or 3 times daily, an individualized meal plan, a program of regular exercise, and frequent blood glucose monitoring combined with the use of algorithms to make insulin and food adjustments based on blood glucose values. We would suggest regular evaluation by a health care team experienced in pediatric diabetes management, as well as using glycohemoglobin determinations several times a year to evaluate success of therapy. Continued education and counselling are essential to maintain the motivation necessary to accomplish the normalization of glucose metabolism which we hope will prevent the microvascular sequelae of diabetes.

References

1 Cahill, G.F.; Etzwiler, D.D.; Frenkel, N.: 'Control' and diabetes. New Engl. J. Med. *294:* 1004–1005 (1976).

2 Sperling, M.A.: Diabetes mellitus. Pediat. Clins N. Am. *26:* 149–169 (1979).

3 Riley, W.J.; Silverstein, J.H.; Rosenbloom, A.L.; Spellar, R.; McCollum, M.H.: Ambulatory diabetes management with pulsed subcutaneous insulin using a portable pump. Clin. Pediat. *19:* 609–614 (1980).

4 Rudolf, M.C.; Ahern, J.A.; Genel, M.; Bates, A.; Harding, P.; Hochstadt, J.; Quintan, P.; Tamborlane, W.V.: Optimal insulin delivery in adolescents with diabetes. Impact of intensive treatment on psychosocial adjustment. Diabetes Care *5:* suppl. 1, pp. 53–57 (1982).

5 Schriffin, A.; Desrosiers, M.; Moffatt, M.; Delmonte, M.M.: Feasibility of strict diabetes control in insulin-dependent diabetic adolescents. J. Pediat. *103:* 522–527 (1983).

6 Daneman, D.; Siminerio, L.; Transue, D.; Betschart, J.; Drash, A.; Becker, D.: The role of self-monitoring of blood glucose in the continued management of children with insulin-dependent diabetes mellitus. Diabetes Care *8:* 1–4 (1985).

7 Topper, E.; Farman, G.; Galatzer, A.; Goldman, J.; Feldberg, D.; Karp, M.; Laron, Z.: Improvement of diabetes control in young diabetics by self blood glucose monitoring; in Laron, Galatzer, Recent progress in medico-social problems in juvenile diabetes (Karger, Basel 1983).

8 Pickup, J.C.; Keen, H.; Parsons, J.A.; Alberti, K.G.M.M.: Continuous subcutaneous insulin infusion. An approach to achieving normoglycemia. Br. med. J. *i:* 204–207 (1978).

9 Tamborlane, W.V.; Sherwin, R.S.; Genel, M.; Felig, P.: Reduction to normal of plasma glucose in juvenile diabetics by subcutaneous administration of insulin with a portable infusion pump. New Engl. J. Med. *300:* 573–578 (1979).

10 Pickup, J.C.; Keen, H.; Parson, J.A.; Alberti, K.G.M.M.; Rowe, A.S.: Continuous subcutaneous insulin infusion: improved blood glucose and intermediary metabolic control in diabetes. Lancet *i:* 1255–1261 (1979).

11 Tamborlane, W.V.; Sherwin, R.S.; Koivisto, V.; Hendler, R.; Genel, M.; Felig, P.: Normalization of the growth hormone and catecholamine response to exercise in juvenile onset diabetics treated with a portable insulin infusion pump. Diabetes *28:* 785–788 (1979).

12 Raskin, P.; Pietri, A.; Unger, R.: Changes in glucagon levels after four to five weeks of glucoregulation by portable insulin infusion pump. Diabetes *28:* 1033–1035 (1979).

13 Pickup, J.C.; Keen, H.; White, M.C.; Parsons, J.A.; Alberti, K.G.M.M.: Long-term continuous subcutaneous insulin infusion in diabetics at home. Lancet *ii:* 870–873 (1979).

14 Tamborlane, W.V.; Sherwin, R.S.; Genel, M.; Felig, P.: Outpatient treatment of juvenile-onset diabetes with a preprogramed portable subcutaneous insulin infusion system. Am. J. Med. *68:* 190–196 (1980).

15 Pietri, A.; Ehle, A.L.; Raskin, P.: Changes in nerve conduction velocity after six weeks of glucoregulation with portable insulin infusion pumps. Diabetes *29:* 668 (1980).

16 White, N.H.; Waltman, S.R.; Krupin, T.; Santiago, J.V.: Reversal of neuropathic and gastrointestinal complications related to diabetes mellitus in adolescents with improved metabolic control. J. Pediat. *99:* 41–45 (1981).

17 Rudolf, M.C.J.; Sherwin, R.S.; Markowitz, R.; Bates, S.E.; Genel, M.; Hochstadt, J.; Tamborlane, W:V.: Effect of intensive insulin treatment on linear growth in the young diabetic patient. J. Pediat. *101:* 333–339 (1982).

18 Koivisto, V.A.; Huttmen, N.-P.; Vierikko, P.: Continuous subcutaneous insulin infusion corrects exercise-induced albuminuria in juvenile diabetes. Br. med. J. *282:* 778–779 (1981).

19 White, N.H.; Waltman, S.R.; Krupin, T.; Santiago, J.V.: Reversal of abnormalities in ocular fluorophotometry in insulin-dependent diabetes after five to nine months of improved metabolic control. Diabetes *31:* 80–85 (1982).

20 Tamborlane, W.V.; Puklin, J.E.; Bergman, M.; Verdonk, C.;

Rudolf, M.C.; Felig, P.; Genel, M.; Sherwin, R.: Long-term improvement of metabolic control with the insulin pump does not reverse diabetic microangiopathy. Diabetes Care *5:* suppl. 1, pp. 58–64 (1982).
21 Viberti, G.C.; Bilows, R.W.; Mackintosh, D.; Bending, J.J.; Keen, H.: Long-term correction of hyperglycemia and progression of renal failure in insulin dependent diabetes. Br. med. J. *286:* 598–609 (1983).
22 Lawson, P.M.; Champion, M.C.; Lanny, C.; Kingsley, R.; White, M.C.; Dupre, J.; Kohner, E.M.: Continuous subcutaneous insulin infusion (CSII) does not prevent progression of proliferative and preproliferative retinopathy. Br. J. Ophthal. *66:* 762–766 (1982).
23 The Kroc Collaborative Study Group: Blood glucose control and the evolution of diabetic retinopathy and albuminuria. New Engl. J. Med. *311:* 365–372 (1984).
24 Rosenstock, J.; Friberg, T.; Raskin, P.: Long-term near normoglycemia slows the progression of diabetic retinopathy. Diabetes *34:* suppl. 1, pp. 159A (1985).
25 Bougneres, P.F.; Landier, F.; Lemmel, C.; Mensire, A.; Chaussain, J.L.: Insulin pump therapy in young children with type 1 diabetes. J. Pediat. *105:* 212–217 (1984).
26 Stewart, C.; Brink, S.; Wentworth, S.: Insulin pump treatment failure in children and adolescents. Pediat. Res. *17:* 515 (1983).
27 Kaye, R.: Research and practice in the treatment of insulin-dependent diabetes: a survey of 53 pediatric diabetologists. Pediatrics *74:* 1079–1085 (1984).
28 Peden, N.R.; Braaten, J.T.; McKendry, J.B.R.: Diabetic ketoacidosis during long-term treatment with continuous subcutaneous insulin infusion. Diabetes Care *7:* 1–5 (1984).
29 Teutsch, S.M.; Herman, W.H.; Dwyer, D.M.; Lane, J.M.: Mortality among diabetic patients using continuous subcutaneous insulin-infusion pumps. New Engl. J. Med. *310:* 361–368 (1984).
30 White, N.H.; Skor, D.A.; Cryer, P.E.; Levandoski, L.A.; Bier, D.M.; Santiago, J.V.: Identification of type I diabetic patients at risk for hypoglycemia during intensive therapy. New Engl. J. Med. *308:* 485–491 (1983).
31 Schriffin, A.; Belmonte, M.: Multiple daily self-glucose monitoring. Its essential role in long-term glucose control in insulin-dependent diabetic patients treated with pump and multiple subcutaneous injections. Diabetes Care *5:* 479–484 (1982).
32 Amercian Diabetes Association Policy Statement: Continuous subcutaneous insulin infusion. Diabetes Care *8:* 516–517 (1985).

Received: December 14, 1985

Georgeanna J. Klingensmith, MD,
The Children's Hospital,
1056 East 19th Avenue,
Denver, CO 80218 (USA)

Pediatrician *12:* 229–235 (1983–85)

0300–1245/85/0124–0229$2.75/0

Techniques for Improving Glucose Control in Type I Diabetes

H. Peter Chase, Barbara Rose, Sandy Hoops, Philip G. Archer, James M. Cribari

Department of Pediatrics, University of Colorado Health Sciences Center, Barbara Davis Center for Childhood Diabetes, Denver, Colo., USA

Key Words. Diabetes · Glycosylated hemoglobin · Glucose control · Intervention · Adolescents

Abstract. Intervention for poor glucose control was attempted in 38 children and adolescents with a mean follow-up time of 3 years. Changing the quantity of insulin or changing the number of injections per day resulted in improvement in 10 of the 21 patients who responded to intervention. Six others responded to a family conference and four responded to a parent temporarily taking over the diabetes management. The presence of a supportive family member living in the home was a major factor in the likelihood of intervention being successful.

Introduction

Type I (insulin-dependent) diabetes is one of the most common diseases of childhood. It is estimated to have a prevalence of three per 1,000 children of 18 years of age or below. Good glucose control is defined as maintaining blood glucose levels as close to normal as possible without causing harm. Glucose control is currently measured by self blood glucose monitoring, glycosylated hemoglobin and the clinical history. Blood glucose control is recognized as being important in relation to growth, acute complications (hypoglycemia and ketoacidosis), pregnancy outcome and some chronic complications (e.g.: neuropathy). It is suspected but not proven to be related to other long-term problems (e.g. retinopathy and nephropathy).

Good glucose control is sometimes difficult to achieve, particularly in adolescents. The purpose of the present paper is to summarize our experience with 38 children and adolescents with poor glucose control who had their baseline visit for the study during 1981, 1982 or 1983. The methods of intervention used in our clinic are presented. The effects of the interventions are evaluated over a mean follow-up time of 3 years.

Methods

All children and adolescents with type I diabetes who had a glycohemoglobin (HbA_1) above 16% when evaluated between 1981 and 1983 and who were at least 6 months after initial diagnosis are included in this report. The total HbA_1 (Isolab, Fast Hemoglobin Test System, with aldimine eliminator to remove the labile fraction) is routinely used in our laboratory; normal values are 6.3–8.2%. The HbA_1 level is usually determined every 3 months at the time of routine clinic visits. For patients in poor control who are seen more frequently the value is determined more often. Clinic records show that we followed approximately 850 people with type I diabetes in 1982 (the middle year): the 38 study patients represent approximately four percent of the clinic population at that time. This percentage of patients in poor control may be high because practitioners often refer difficult cases to us while continuing to follow less difficult cases in their own offices. Our approach toward the routine clinical management of children and adolescents with type I diabetes has been presented elsewhere [1, 2].

The methods of intervention, listed in the order usually followed, are shown in table I. This order sometimes varied; for example, some people began working with the psychologist earlier, whereas others did not see her until later. Although all methods of intervention were available to all patients, some patients improved at an earlier time (e.g., after increasing or decreasing the insulin dosage) so that all means of intervention were not needed, nor were they attempted. In addition, some patients refused one or more suggested interventions (e.g., frequent phone contact, frequent

Table I. Methods of intervention

1	Increase insulin dosage (> 10%)
2	Change in number of injections per day
3	New emphasis on self blood glucose monitoring
4	Frequent telephone monitoring
5	Frequent visits to clinic
6	Psychologic help
7	Family conference
8	Parents taking over management

Table II. Age distributions of the study and the general clinic population

Age	Study population	General clinic population
< 5 years	0	5%
5 years – 9 years 11 months	0	18%
10 years – 12 years 11 months	26%	21%
13 years – 15 years 11 months	53%	28%
16 years – 18 years 11 months	21%	28%

clinic visits, regular use of self-blood glucose monitoring, seeing the psychologist, etc.)

Glucose control was arbitrarily defined by the HbA_1 level, with a value of > 16.0% being poor, 13.0–15.9% being fair, 11.0–12.9% being good and < 11.0% being excellent. The value of 10.9% is 1.5 times our normal mean and does not represent perfect control. It is unknown if a value below 11% is good enough to prevent sequelae.

The first time the HbA_1 value was above 16% was taken as the zero time for each patient. The value approximately 12 months later was the 1-year value, 24 months later the 2-year value, etc. When more than one value was available in a given year of follow-up, the mean of the last two values for that 12 month period was used in classifying glycemic control for that year.

Our definition of a meaningful change in the glycohemoglobin value, indicating the effectiveness of a method of intervention, was taken to be a decrease of more than 1.8 percentage points. The mean glycohemoglobin value for our entire clinic population decreased from 12.7 to 11.7% during this time, so that a decrease of one percent might have occurred without specific intervention. Secondly, the error factor for our laboratory in the HbA_1 determination (multiple samples, same day or same sample on multiple days) is ± 0.4% (± 1 SD).

Most of the methods of intervention (table I) are self explanatory. The 'new emphasis on self blood glucose monitoring' was counted only if the person previously had not been doing any regular self blood glucose determinations and was then willing to make results available from at least two tests per week. An 'increase in the insulin dosage' was counted only if there was an increase of at least 10% of the dose at the time of the high initial glycohemoglobin. 'Frequent telephone monitoring' was credited if the person was willing to call in testing results to the health care provider at least once weekly. All phone calls were documented with phone encounter records. 'Frequent clinic visits' was credited if the person came into the clinic at least once monthly. 'Psychologic help' was credited if the person made at least three visits to the psychologist or social worker outside of routine clinic appointments. The 'family conference' consisted of both parents (or parent-substitutes) and the patient and siblings sitting together in a conference room with the doctor and/or child health associate (pediatric physician assistant), the nurse, the dietitian and the psychologist or social worker. The importance of good glucose control was discussed at the conference and a plan outlined for helping the patient to achieve good control. The 'parents taking over management' meant that the parents would give or closely observe all injections and do or closely supervise all blood testing.

Results

The age distributions of the 38 study patients and of our general clinic population are shown in table II. Fifty three percent of the study patients were between ages 13 years and 15 years 11 months, whereas only 28% of the general clinic population were in this age group. There were no study patients under 10 years of age, compared to 22% of the general clinic population in this age range. The study group consisted of 15 males (40%) and 23 females (60%). This was similar to our general clinic population of 46% males and 54% females. Thirty of the patients were of Anglo background, three were Black and five were of Mexican-American descent. This ethnic distribution was similar to that of our general clinic population.

The mean (± 1 SD) starting glycohemoglobin for all 38 subjects was 18.2 (± 1.6) %. The mean (± 1 SD) value was 13.1 (± 2.3)% at the time of the last follow-up (mean = 36.5 months, range 11–52 months). During this period, all patients improved their glycohemoglobin value to at least the 'fair' range (13.0–15.9%) on at least one occasion. After 1 year, follow-up was available for all 38 patients (fig. 1). Twenty five (66%) showed improvement in their glycohemoglobin level with one in the excellent range; 13 were in the poor range. At year 2, follow-up was available for 34 people; three were in the excellent range and nine in the poor range. After 3 years, follow-up was available for 32 people; four were in the excellent range and five in the poor range.

When the glycohemoglobin values from throughout the study period for each individual patient were plotted on a time graph, three distinct patterns or types of improvement could be distinguished:

Group 1 = consistent improvement (15 people)
Group 2 = inconsistent improvement (18 people)
Group 3 = no improvement (5 people).

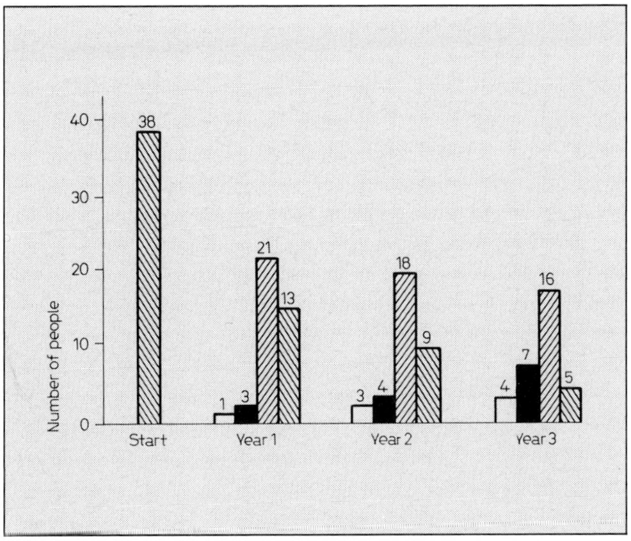

Fig. 1. Changes in glucose control in the 3 years following intervention. The numbers above each bar represent the number of patients in that group. ▧ = Poor control ($HbA_1 > 16.0\%$); ▨ = fair control (HbA_1 13.0–15.9%); ■ = good control (HbA_1 = 11.0–12.9%); □ = excellent control ($HbA_1 < 11\%$).

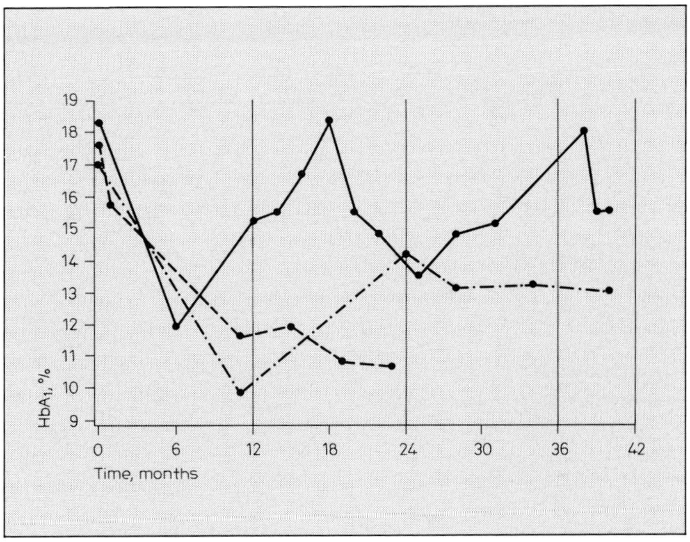

Fig. 2. Typical graphs representing the three types of improvement: consistent improvement (– – –), inconsistent improvement (– · – · –) and no improvement (——).

These divisions were made arbitrarily by visual inspection of graphs. Group 1 patients showed a consistent improvement in their glycohemoglobin values. Group 2 patients fluctuated widely during the period of study but tended to show improvement. Group 3 patients remained in or near the poor range throughout the study. This may seem quite arbitrary, but three professionals (HPC, BR and PGA) had no difficulty agreeing on each case. 'Consistent improvement' and 'no improvement' were easily spotted, and the intermediate cases were arrived at by exclusion. Figure 2 shows a typical graph of each group.

An effort was made to determine whether simple objective measures (specifically, the overall slope, parametric and nonparametric correlation coefficients) could be used, either singularly or in combination, to distinguish one type of curve from another. While some discrimination could be achieved using slopes and correlations, it was not nearly as clear-cut as the overall gestalt perceived from viewing the graph.

The initial mean (±1 SD) glycohemoglobin values were similar for all three groups: group 1 = 18.3 ± 1.3%, group 2 = 18.3 ± 1.7% and group 3 = 18.0 ± 2.3%. The final mean (±1 SD) glycohemoglobin value for each of the 3 groups was: group 1 = 11.4 ± 1.4%, group 2 = 13.7 ± 1.6% and group 3 = 16.3 ± 2.1%.

An effective intervention was defined as one which resulted in a fall in HbA_1 by 1.9 or more percentage points (see Methods) in the 6 months after introducing the intervention. When the effectiveness of the various methods of intervention was analyzed, there were two distinct groups (table III). Group A consisted of 21 people (55%) where a clear temporal relationship was demonstrated between the onset of an intervention and a subsequently lowered glycohemoglobin value. The mean (±1 SD) decrease in the glycohemoglobin value for group A patients in the 6 months after intervention was 5.0 (± 2.6) percentage points (range: 1.9–12.6 points). The mean (±1 SD) decrease in the 12 months following intervention was 5.4 (± 2.3) percentage points (range: 1.9–12.6).The greatest decrease (12.6 percentage points in three months) was for a 15-year-old boy who responded to a family conference which included another method of intervention (having an aunt take over all insulin injections). The boy readily admitted to not taking his insulin when he wanted to get out of his living situation.

Group B consisted of 17 people (45%) for whom there was no apparent association between an attempt at intervention and a decrease in the glycohemoglobin level. While some of the individuals in group B did improve in glycohemoglobin level, the improvement did not meet the criterion of a reduction of 1.9 or more percentage

Table III. Frequency of use of methods of intervention

	Methods of intervention[1]							
	1	2	3	4	5	6	7	8
Group A (21 people)								
Accepted implementation	10 (48%)	12 (57%)	11 (52%)	8 (38%)	12 (57%)	16 (76%)	12 (57%)	12 (58%)
Refused to initiate	0	0	10 (48%)	8 (38%)	6 (29%)	3 (14%)	0	4 (18%)
Not indicated or not offered	11 (52%)	9 (43%)	0	5 (24%)	3 (14%)	2 (10%)	9 (43%)	5 (24%)
Group B (17 people)								
Accepted implementation	11 (65%)	13 (76%)	6 (35%)	11 (65%)	10 (59%)	8 (47%)	9 (53%)	5 (29%)
Refused to initiate	0	1 (6%)	9 (53%)	6 (35%)	7 (41%)	9 (53%)	1 (6%)	9 (53%)
Not indicated or not offered	6 (35%)	3 (18%)	2 (12%)	0	0	0	7 (41%)	3 (18%)

[1] Methods of intervention are the same as in table I.

points within 6 months of introducing a specific intervention.

The methods of intervention most strongly related to improvement of the glycohemoglobin values in the 21 group A people are shown in table IV. These were determined by listing the interventions and noting which resulted in a fall in the glycohemoglobin value of 1.9 or more percentage points in the ensuing 6 months. The numbers add up to more than 21 because more than one method of intervention was used simultaneously for 4 of the patients. The three methods of intervention that were associated most frequently with a decrease in the glycohemoglobin value were: increasing the insulin dosage by at least 10% to an average of 1.1 U/kg body weight (5 people), changing the number of injections per day (5 people) and having a family conference (6 people). There were another 5 group A patients who did not respond to increasing their insulin dosage, but who did respond to another intervention (table III). There were also 11 patients in group B who did not respond to increasing the insulin dosage, so that the total success rate was 5 of 21 patients. The improvement in the 5 patients was sustained after follow-up periods of 8, 13, 15, 43 and 48 months. The mean initial and final (at the time of last follow-up) glycohemoglobin values for the five patients responding to increased insulin dosage were 17.5 and 12.1%, respectively. The mean decrease at the time of last follow-up was 5.4% (range 1.8–8.4 points). All five people were in the 'good' control range (11.0–12.9%) at the time of last follow-up.

Among the five patients who showed a lowering of the glycohemoglobin value by 1.9 or more percentage points following a change in the number of daily insulin injections, four were changed from two to one injection daily. All four admitted to missing the evening injection on one or more occasions per week. They were changed to the same total dose of insulin, given only once daily. One other person who was on one injection per day at the time of her initial high glycohemoglobin value showed improvement after being changed to twice daily insulin injections. Four of these five patients were thereafter able to sustain their improved glycohemoglobin levels by 1.9 or more percentage points below the initially elevated value. The fifth person improved for a period of 14 months, but then lapsed into her previous poor control. The mean initial and final (at last follow-up) glycohemoglobin values for the four patients showing sustained improvement were 17.3 and 10.5%, respectively. The mean decrease for these four patients was 6.8% (range 4.7–8.9 points). Two of the four were in the 'good' control range and two were in the 'excellent' range (< 11%). The glycohemoglobin level of the fifth person fell from an initial value of 18.1% to a level of 8.6% 5 months after changing to one injection per day. She had a level of 11.8% after 8 months. She was then temporarily lost to follow-up but returned with a value of 17.8% 14 months after her initial improvement. Twenty other patients had changes in the number of insulin injections per day but did not show subsequent improvement in their glycohemoglobin levels.

Six of the 21 patients having a family conference showed a decline in the glycohemoglobin of 1.9 or more percentage points in the following 6 months (table IV). In two of these six, however, the intervention was combined with an adult taking over the diabetes management. In a third person, the family conference initiated other interventions from table I, all of which may have contributed to better control. Three of the six patients who improved as a result of the family conference were able to maintain their improved glucose control for follow-up periods of 13, 15 and 23 months. The mean initial and final (at last follow-up) glycohemoglobin values for these three were 18.0 and 10.8%, respectively. Two of the three were in the 'excellent' control range and the third was in the 'good' range at the time of last follow-up. The other three patients improved and then assumed variable courses: one improved on three occasions but twice relapsed (HbA_1 of 11.7% at last follow-up); one improved, relapsed and then again improved (HbA_1 of 12.9% at last follow-up); the final person improved and then relapsed (HbA_1 of 14.8% at last follow-up). A total of 21 patients had family conferences, so that this method of intervention was not successful for 15 patients. With one girl, two family conferences, held 3 months apart were associated with a negative influence in both instances, as manifested by subsequent elevations in her glycohemoglobin levels.

Both individuals who showed improvement after psychological intervention showed some worsening of their glycohemoglobin levels initially (one at 2 months and the other after 3 months), prior to periods of prolonged improvement.

Sustained improvement occurred more often in group A patients (57%), where improvement followed an intervention, than in the group B patients (18%) where there was no apparent association between intervention and improved glycemic control (table V). Likewise, 'no improvement' was seen more frequently in the group B patients (24%) than in the group A patients (5%). Over one-half of the families in group B refused to initiate 'psychological help' and 'parents taking over management' when these interventions were requested (table III). In contrast, refusal rates were 14 and 18%, respectively, for these two items when requested of the families in group A.

Table IV. Method of intervention primarily contributing to improvement

Method	Number of patients improving	Total number who accepted the method
Increase in insulin dosage (by 10% or more)	5	21
Changing the number of injections per day	5	25
Family conference (only as intervention)	6	21
Parents taking over management	4	17
Psychologic help	2	24
New emphasis on self blood glucose monitoring	2	17
Frequent telephone monitoring	1	19
Frequents visits to clinics	0	22

Table V. The effects of intervention or the degree of improvement

Response group	Group A	Group B
Group 1	12 (57)	3 (18)
Group 2	8 (38)	10 (59)
Group 3	1 (5)	4 (24)

Figures represent number of patients with percentage in parentheses.

Discussion

This study evaluated methods of intervention routinely used in our clinic for patients with poor glucose control. A follow-up time of 3 years for 32 of the 38 patients showed long-term improvement in 27 patients (84%). Two methods of intervention, a change in the quantity of insulin and a change in the number of injections per day, were judged to be a primary component in contributing to improvement in 10 of the 21 people (48%) who showed improvement as a result of intervention. This represented 26% of the total study population of 38 people. These methods of intervention are relatively simple and can be carried out by a pediatrician without the involvement of a diabetes team. They should be given primary consideration in any patient with poor glucose control.

The family conference requires considerable time and effort from the family and the health care team, but is considered the next most effective intervention resulting in improvement. We try to approach the family conference in a concerned and caring way, and not in a threatening manner. We tell all families that our purpose is to work with them to improve the patient's glucose control. At the end of the conference, we give the family a sheet with the objective information and the clearly outlined plan.

It is likely that some of the interventions resulted in a cumulative positive effect even though there was not an obvious subsequent lowering of the glycohemoglobin value. For example, working with the psychologist may have helped the patient in placing frequent phone calls to the physician or in increasing the use of self blood glucose monitoring, or possibly, in accepting the diabetic condition and learning to live with it more effectively. It was impossible to measure the subtle effects of some of the interventions. It is likely, however, that they were important.

Since this study began, we have realized that most – if not all – children and teenagers who have glycohemoglobin levels above 16%, and who have a reported insulin dose of approximately 1 U/kg body weight, are frequently missing insulin injections. In recent reports, other investigators have also noted that many children [4] and adults [5] who present with recurrent DKA are missing insulin injections. *Golden* et al. [4] noted, 'In 44 patients with a history of recurrent DKA, insulin omission was documented in 31'. We now confront the patient with the statement, 'It is impossible to have a glycohemoglobin level that high and not be forgetting some of your shots. How many shots per week do you usually forget?' The most frequent answer is, 'One or two per week'. One 15-year-old boy admitted he only *took* one or two shots per week! If the patient usually forgets the evening dose, changing to one morning injection per day may be the best intervention. A controlled study has now been initiated in our clinic to evaluate the effectiveness of changing to one injection per day in patients who present with high glycohemoglobin levels. If morning and evening injections are both intermittently missed, 'parents taking over management' (intervention 8 in table I) is usually necessary for a month or longer, if a supportive parent is available in the home. During this time the patient often realizes how much better he/she feels when receiving the insulin regularly. The parents can gradually gain insight into the problem as they observe the fall in glycohemoglobin when they give all the injections.

The age distribution differed from our general clinic population in that no person in the study group was under age 10 years (22% of our general clinic population is under age 10). Parents are usually responsible for diabetes management in the younger child; also, adolescent rebellion has not yet begun. In contrast, over half of the study population was between ages 13 years and 15 years 11 months, compared to only 28% of the general clinic population. The early teen years appear to be a time of high-risk for poor diabetes control.

The use of the glycohemoglobin value to measure glucose control is not an inclusive measure of overall diabetes control [3]. For example, a child with a very low glycohemoglobin value who is having severe, potentially brain-damaging hypoglycemic episodes is certainly not in good overall diabetes control. The present study dealt with the problem of sustained hyperglycemia rather than the entire range of problems associated with diabetes.

A subjective opinion was made by three members of the clinical staff as to whether each patient had a supportive family member living in the home who 'cared about the person with diabetes and was willing to participate in the day-to-day management of the diabetes'. The results were then examined in relation to the patient's placement into group 1, group 2 or group 3 over the 3 years (as in fig. 2). A supportive parent had been judged present for 14 of the 15 in group 1, seven of 18 in group 2 and 0 of five in group 3. A supportive parent in the home may be the most important predictor in regards to whether intervention will be successful in improving a child or adolescent's diabetes control.

Schiffrin et al. [6] have emphasized intensive insulin therapy and continuous subcutaneous insulin infusion as methods for improving care. The patients in their study started with a mean glycohemoglobin level of 13%, however, which is quite different than starting at a level above 16% as in the present study. No interventions work when the patients are noncompliant unless a dramatic change occurs in the patient, such as sometimes happens with the onset of complications, or unless someone else takes over the diabetes management for a period of time. In the present study, if changing the dose of insulin was not a successful intervention, it was essential to have a supportive parent in the home. This parent might have helped to supervise or to give injections, to see that the blood sugars were being done accurately, or to be certain that contacts were made with appropriate members of the diabetes team. Without the supportive parent, success was unlikely to occur.

Acknowledgement

This research was supported by grant No. HD 14985 from the National Institute of Child Health and Human Development, and by a grant (RR 69) from the General Clinical Research Centers Programs of the Division of Research Resources, National Institutes of Health.

References

1 Chase, H.P.: Avoiding the short- and long-term complications of juvenile diabetes. Pediat. Rev. *7:* 138–149 (1985).
2 Chase, H.P.: Understanding insulin dependent diabetes; 5th ed. (Herschfeld Press, Denver 1983).
3 Chase, H.P.: Monitoring glucose control and use of a diabetes control index in insulin-dependent diabetes mellitus. Pediatr. Ann. *12:* 643–650 (1983).
4 Golden, M.P.; Herrold, A.J.; Orr, D.P.: An approach to prevention of recurrent diabetic ketoacidosis in the pediatric population. J. Pediat. *107:* 195–200 (1985).
5 Fulop, M.: Recurrent diabetic ketoacidosis. Am. J. Med. *78:* 54–60 (1985).
6 Schiffrin, A.D.; Desrosiers, M.; Aleyassine, H.; Belmonte, M.M.: Intensified insulin therapy in the type I diabetic adolescent: a controlled trial. Diabetes Care *7:* 107–113 (1984).

Received: December 19, 1985

H. Peter Chase, MD,
Department of Pediatrics,
University of Colorado Health Sciences Center,
Barbara Davis Center for Childhood Diabetes,
4200 East 9th Avenue,
Box B-140,
Denver, CO 80262 (USA)

Author Index

Subject Index

S. Karger · Medical and Scientific Publishers · Basel · München · Paris · London · New York · New Delhi · Singapore · Tokyo · Sydney

Drug Dosage
The authors and the publisher have exerted every effort to ensure that drug selection and dosage set forth in this text are in accord with current recommendations and practice at the time of publication. However, in view of ongoing research, changes in government regulations, and the constant flow of information relating to drug therapy and drug reactions, the reader is urged to check the package insert for each drug for any change in indications and dosage and for added warnings and precautions. This is particularly important when the recommended agent is a new and/or infrequently employed drug.

Printed in Switzerland by Thür AG Offsetdruck, Pratteln
ISBN 3–8055–4400–6

Vol. 12, 1983-85

Pediatrician

International Journal of Child and Adolescent Health

Founded 1858 as 'Jahrbuch für Kinderheilkunde und physische Erziehung', continued as 'Annales Paediatrici' (1938–1966), 'Pediatric Research' (1967–1970) and 'Paediatrician' (1972–1982)

KARGER

S. Karger · Medical and Scientific Publishers · Basel · München · Paris · London · New York · New Delhi · Singapore · Tokyo · Sydney

Drug Dosage

The authors and the publisher have exerted every effort to ensure that drug selection and dosage set forth in this text are in accord with current recommendations and practice at the time of publication. However, in view of ongoing research, changes in government regulations, and the constant flow of information relating to drug therapy and drug reactions, the reader is urged to check the package insert for each drug for any change in indications and dosage and for added warnings and precautions. This is particularly important when the recommended agent is a new and/or infrequently employed drug.

Printed in Switzerland by Thür AG Offsetdruck, Pratteln

Contents Vol. 12, 1983-85

No. 1

Violent Deaths in Childhood and Adolescence

No. 2-3

Eating Disorders: Obesity, Anorexia nervosa, and Bulimia in Childhood and Adolescence

No. 4

Diabetes in Childhood and Adolescence

Medicine and Sport Science (ISSN 0254-5020), **Vol. 20**
Series Editor: M. Hebbelinck, Brussels

Growth, Health and Fitness of Teenagers

Longitudinal Research in International Perspective
Volume Editor: H.C.G. Kemper, Amsterdam

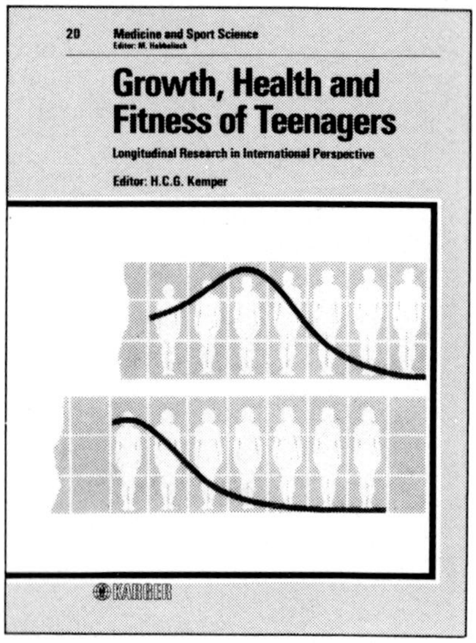

The complete report of a study certain to interest a wide audience of sports physicians, coaches and trainers, school physicians, physical educators, psychologists and dieticians.

This book describes the design, methods, and results of a major longitudinal study conducted to elicit information on the growth, health, and physical fitness of teenagers in Holland. Multidisciplinary in design, the study involved numerous and repeated tests of mental and physical variables in more than 600 school children between the ages of 12 and 18 years. Among its many goals, the study attempted to detect changes in habitual patterns of food intake and physical activity and to determine the extent to which these changes are reflected in altered health.

The book opens with a survey of longitudinal studies of adolescent growth and development carried out since 1900. An analysis of strengths and weaknesses of these studies is then used to explain the methodology and goals of the present work. Chapters provide full details on study design, subjects and procedures, including a thorough explanation of all methods used to measure and assess physical and psychosocial status and changes, eating and smoking habits, and habitual physical activity.

The results of the study are then presented and discussed in a total of 10 chapters. Results cover growth changes of height and weight, patterns of biological development, changes in body build and composition, and how these changes differ according to sex. Other chapters discuss the results of functional measurements of motor performance and maximal aerobic power and compare these results with data recorded in the world literature. The remaining chapters report findings on cardiovascular risk indicators, developmental changes in personality and sociometric status, and changes in eating habits and daily physical activity.

Contents

Medicine and Sport Science, Vol. 20
Growth, Health and Fitness of Teenagers
Longitudinal Research in International Perspective
Volume Editor: H.C.G. Kemper, Amsterdam
XII + 204 p., 95 fig., 24 tab., hard cover, 1985
SFr. 116.– / DM 139.– / US $ 64.50
DM / US $ prices subject to change
ISBN 3-8055-4042-6

KARGER

KI 85064